DESIGNING THE
OPEN NURSING HOME

COMMUNITY DEVELOPMENT SERIES

Series Editor: Richard P. Dober, AIP

CDS / 27

DESIGNING THE OPEN NURSING HOME

Joseph A. Koncelik

The Ohio State University

Dowden, Hutchinson & Ross, Inc.
STROUDSBURG, PENNSYLVANIA

Copyright © 1976 by **Dowden, Hutchinson & Ross, Inc.**
Community Development Series, Volume 27
Library of Congress Catalog Card Number: 76–11010
ISBN: 0–87933–236–0

78 77 76 5 4 3 2 1
Manufactured in the United States of America.

LIBRARY OF CONGRESS CATALOGING IN PUBLICATION DATA

Koncelik, Joseph A.
    Designing the open nursing home.
    (Community development series/27)
    Bibliography
    Includes index.
    1. Nursing homes—Design and construction. I. Title.
RA997.K66   725'.56   76–11010
ISBN 0–87933–236–0

SERIES EDITOR'S PREFACE

The Community Development Series is intended to facilitate the exchange of information, expert advice, and experience among professionals concerned with the built environment. CDS publications include state-of-the-art books, reference works, handbooks, and manuals. They are written for planners, architects, landscape architects, engineers, and those in related disciplines who may find benefits in having such knowledge in a readily convenient format.

Community here is defined in the broadest sense and includes the diverse places that support human activities in all their manifestations. They range in scale from a family room to the metropolis. Obviously, such places vary in size, function, configuration, and detailed attributes; accordingly, planning and design methodologies that are used in shaping these places will differ in approach and realization.

In working with community as defined, CDS is not bounded by traditional theory, nor does it presume to establish a philosophic framework for all professional practices. However, there are some themes that do identify CDS books conceptually. These propositions include: active user and client involvement in problem defining and problem solving; systematic searching out of patterns, relationships, and behavioral settings as a prelude to design; a high regard for physical interdependence of communities; ecological ethics; and an interest in not just finding appropriate solutions, but also in establishing ways and means for having those solutions implemented.

From time to time CDS books will appeal to and serve a larger audience than just the professions. It will do so because the subject matter will help the owner, user, and manager of the built environment to become more aware of issues, possibilities, and techniques. The books will be organized so that participation and involvement can move from the rhetoric of good intentions to the reality of dealing with substantive matters in comprehensive detail.

Joseph A. Koncelik's is one such book. It is written to serve all those concerned with planning, designing, and operating open nursing homes. These environments shelter an ever-increasing part of our population. In the main, they have not been beneficial environments, not so much because good-willed people have avoided their responsibilities, but because definitive research was not available to influence and guide their architecture. That void is now filled with this comprehensive treatise.

By approaching his subject systematically, Koncelik

provides the novice and the knowledgeable with insights, concepts, and executed examples that will raise the quality of these important places. The material is also arranged so that alternative ideas—possibly better ones—can be discovered by others who will profit by following his lines of inquiry. Using this approach, both method and content should have a long shelf life, thus making his book a basic reference work in the field.

It is our hope to publish additional books singularly focused. By strengthening our knowledge of behavioral settings as a design influence on specialized environments, we strengthen an important root source in contemporary architectural theory and practice.

Richard P. Dober, AIP

PREFACE

Designing the modern nursing home is an extremely complex and time-consuming task involving the expertise of many professional disciplines, as well as the input of community and potential patients—if the job is to be done well. Often the complexities dominate, and the excessive burden of integrating the tremendous number of pieces of the problem forces expedient choices at the level where concentrated design effort should be brought to bear—the spaces accessible to the people who must live in the setting.

The typical planning and design process begins with decisions about funding, regulatory structures, organizational patterns, and specific designations of building programs, which have really little bearing on the environment that will be created in the end. Unfortunately, as a result of current planning and design practice, in too many cases the environments are an afterthought.

The situation is actually dangerous. In just two decades, nursing homes have gone from being small converted dwelling units averaging about 26 occupants to campus facilities sometimes housing over 1000 people. In a very short time, this society has developed a means by which infirm older people are brought together in large numbers under one roof and treated,

both in terms of their infirmities and their style of life, through programs. While the nursing home has become safer, cleaner, more professional, and more accountable, it has also become an important economic, social, and psychological presence in the life of 1 million older Americans.

In the beginning parts of this book, the reader will find that, during the massive building effort which took place over the past two decades, there was no clear concept of what to build. In other words, America is currently living with a legacy of institutional settings constructed in ignorance. The largest percentage of environments succeed because of the efforts of nursing home personnel to make the setting as much a responsive and "prosthetic" environment as possible.

Although there is little likelihood that a new construction boom will result from the research conducted on institutional settings since the 1950s, there should be a tremendous effort to change and refurbish existing structures, as well as to build new environments with a greater consciousness of the needs of the older people who will reside or are residing in the nursing home.

It would be erroneous to conclude that there is

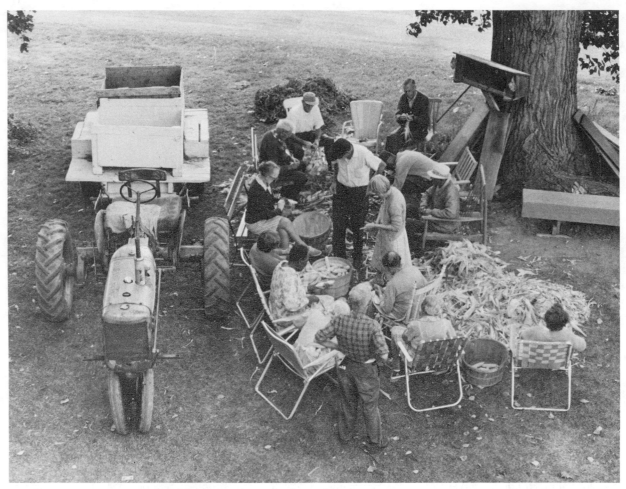

Shucking corn at a county home and farm. (Photo: David O. Watkins.)

s¯me malevolent force present preventing good design of institutional settings and the furnishings chosen to outfit the setting. There is no blame to be leveled at any one professional group or at the consortia of professionals who work to put together the physical environment. The reason that there are so many poorly designed institutional settings is that design did not penetrate, as an activity, to the level where it touches the lives of the residents of the facility.

Today, the architect is an assembler of parts who must work terribly fast on complex problems so that a project is completed within a predetermined time period with as little difficulty as possible. Thus, the building will seldom be experimental, nor will the architect have time to become informed in depth about the nature of the problem to be tackled. The most that can be done in the majority of design projects is to investigate those previous answers and work with those sources which will provide ready and proven answers. All design is eclectic on a philosophic level, but the design process in institutional building is totally eclectic, right down to the choice of hardware.

Keeping this in mind, there should be no mystery as to why mistakes are duplicated when there is no ready evidence of previous mistakes or poor choices of materials and hardware. If this lack of information seems to be the rule at the detail level, there is even less "source information" about the planning and designing for living in these settings at the microenvironmental level. While the design process is frequently efficient in terms of synthesizing information about general layout, plans, facades, and mechanical detailing, very little attention is given at all to the design of the actual living space. There is no time in the design process, as the situation presently exists, to devote effort to the surroundings that will directly affect the lives of the residents. This seems almost shocking, but after the plans have been generated and the overall specifications worked out, the architect's services are usually terminated. Someone else other than the architect will "design" the interior of the building. Sometimes an interior designer is chosen or, if there is real design consciousness, the architect's interior design staff is utilized to make selections for the interior outfitting of the building. However, very frequently an administrator may actually be responsible for the interior setting; in some cases, even the occupational therapist is given the responsibility of choosing the interior decor materials, hardware, and furnishings.

Thus, the situation surrounding the creation of the most important aspect of the environment, the design of the accessible space, is not really a design process at all. Nursing homes seem highly institutional and largely barren of stimulating design content because (1) the largest percentage were built before there was a good working body of knowledge on what should be built in the first place; (2) architects have to work

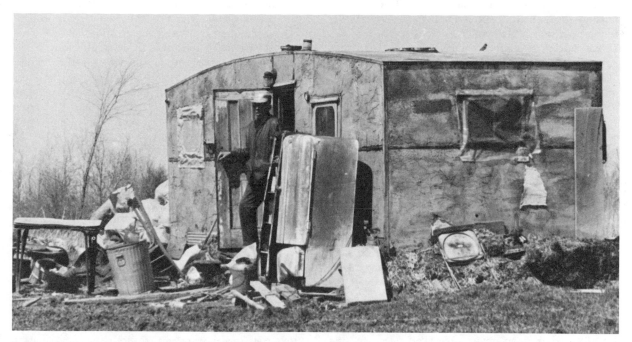

Rural residence of an elderly man. The living conditions of many indigent rural elderly people are terrible. Although upgrading of housing is not a rationale for institutionalization, a high percentage of these elderly people have serious nutrition and health problems. For many there are few alternatives outside of moving into an institutional setting. (Photo: David O. Watkins.)

too fast and, in so doing, do not get involved in the microenvironmental detailing of the setting; (3) in any case, their services are often concluded prior to microenvironmental design and the task is delegated to someone without design expertise.

How can the situation be rectified? It is impossible to really say how better design and a better design process can be injected into the present situation. One small step is the creation of source information that is useful at the time the design program commences and through its duration. This book is an attempt to be a source about the microenvironment. It is not a "cookbook." This book is not written to delineate exactly what the shape and character of any given nursing home should be. It is an attempt to provide information on the inhabitants and their problems, the character of accessibility, and possible alternatives for outfitting the interior environment. The book is also an attempt to provoke a fundamental change in attitude about the elderly infirm and the nursing home environment. Openness, as it is defined, is the provision of as many apertures for getting out of the setting as there are for getting in. It is also a strong desire to have the heavy and oppressive health care atmosphere of the nursing home become far more recessive and to have the residential nature of the facility emerge and predominate.

While the design process may not change, at least not very rapidly, there should be an honest recognition of where the process is weak and who is responsible for the design of much of the internal environment. If an administrator, nurse, or occupational therapist is going to be involved in the design process, then they should try to recognize some of the qualitative aspects of design decision making, which they cannot become aware of without source material. In this sense, this text has been written with as little jargon as possible to reach the greatest possible audience.

In conclusion, there is a need to be realistic about the nursing home—its potential and its limitations. The nursing home, in all its variations, cannot be transformed into an environmental panacea for the nation's elderly people. To be sure, the ratio of those over that magical age of 65 who must confront institutional life is a small fraction of the total popula-tion. Yet, in terms of financial cost there is a great need to make sure that these environments are the very best they can be. The nursing home is only one part of a health care system with many parts. The nursing home is not the end of a steady linear progression of decline, but a kind of energizer in a continuous health care loop. To make it what it should be, attitudes of hopefulness about the nursing home must be developed for old people. While design expertise should be brought to bear as intensively at the microenvironmental level as possible, the design process is becoming participatory. Perhaps who designs is less important than the final product. The aging infirm have lived with too many mistakes made with much good intention.

ACKNOWLEDGMENTS

The author is greatly indebted to many people, who not only cooperated in research projects with him or provided insights at critical times on various projects, but also helped to change his attitudes, allowing him to become more receptive to concepts about design from nondesigners and to see more clearly the need for an expanded frame of reference for all design activity. Foremost in this large group of people are Edward R. Ostrander, Ph.D., and Lorraine H. Snyder. In 1970, these two bright and creative behavioral scientists joined in mutual cooperation with the author on the first of three research projects dealing with the evaluation of the design of nursing homes. Over the next three years, this team, along with the cooperation of some extremely talented students, experienced one of the most painful, distressing, and arduous periods in their lives. What was embarked upon blithely as an interdisciplinary venture became a lesson in the distances between professions.

However, while the pain was great, the productivity was greater. Many acknowledge today that the reports, articles, and presentations generated, as well as the techniques used in the research process and analysis, were some of the most provocative and useful materials devised. Indeed, without the microenvironmental information generated at that time, this book would not be possible. Fortunately, Dr. Ostrander is currently documenting the entire project at Cornell

University and will make the summary available as a publication.

The author also wishes to thank Professor Rose Steidl for her cooperation and guidance during the projects at Cornell, and Edward Matey, graduate assistant, who helped to formulate much of the specifications on seating and generated an early draft of the much needed information on the physiological aspects of aging.

Also at Cornell, the guidance of Professor Philip Taietz, Professor Katherine Visnyei, and Ms. Arpie Shelton is greatly appreciated. Their long experience in gerontology was an important force in allowing the author an exceedingly fast development time and orientation to the problems of aging.

Support for the research conducted at Cornell could only have been obtained because of the foresight and faith of David Knapp, dean of the College of Human Ecology; Professor Joseph Carreiro, chairman of the Department of Design and Environmental Analysis; and Lucinda Noble, associate dean of the College of Human Ecology.

Many talented people assisted in the various projects over time and especially in the three projects at Cornell. Most notably, five students who participated in the research at Cornell and helped develop the concept of the project, the data-collection methods, and the behavior mapping graphics were Karen Brandhorst, Susan Jaye, Susan Marko, John Kelsey, and Robert Steinbugler. A sixth student, Louis Scolnick, developed a system of graphic symbols for the behavior mapping illustrations. Karen Brandhorst and Robert Steinbugler helped set up a method to create the illustrations and to project the initial data during observation sessions in the settings.

Appreciation is also expressed for the work of Linda Nelson, graduate assistant, Allen MacManes, and Lindsey Alley, who were extremely helpful assisting with data analysis. Thanks also to Gail Cohen and June MacManes, who were so helpful in translating material to typed records, transcribing tape recordings, and moving the projects.

During this same period of time, others outside Cornell University were extremely helpful. Mr. Lawrence Larson, vice-president of the Isabella Geriatric Center and his staff were extremely helpful during the re-

search phases. Also, at Syracuse University, Walter Beattie, director of the All-University Gerontology Center; Darrel Slover, assistant professor of Social Work, and Kermit Schooler, dean of the College of Social Work were all very generous with their comments, advice, and experience sharing.

One difficulty encountered in conducting research projects, as pointed out in Pirsig's insightful *Zen and the Art of Motorcycle Maintenance*, is that the generation of one hypothesis within the context of the scientific method begets the generation of an infinite number of hypotheses that follow. The creation of knowledge is really the creation of more questions. So, too, the experiences of the author in research were such that ever more research had to be conducted in order to achieve greater completeness. However, environmental studies cannot be conducted as research without development. The problem inherent in such an approach is that the conditions under which design is conducted are constantly evolving. Therefore, information on specific environments can become outdated before it is ever used.

It seemed necessary, after the initial experiences gathered in the environmental evaluation projects, to shift the frame of reference to research and development and with this came the shift to Ohio State University. Much of the material in specification form reached developmental stages at Ohio State University through work conducted by the author in conjunction with Dwight Bonner, assistant professor. Professor Bonner's undergraduate students undertook a significant project leading to the development of more refined specifications and prototype room configurations for a new nursing home at the First Community Village in Columbus, Ohio. Other students working with the author further established other product and specification development, which made a substantial contribution to this book. Of importance is Richard Kieselbach's work on lighting, Bruce McPherson's work on food service systems and product development in this area, and Michael French's experimentation in seated comfort and profile analysis.

Colleagues who have lent a great deal of encouragement and assistance both in the author's research and this document are numerous. Professor Leon Pastalan of the University of Michigan, M. Powell Lawton,

Ph.D., research director at the Philadelphia Geriatric Center, and Thomas Byerts, director of environment and design research in the Gerontological Society, have been instrumental in moving the substance of the author's work through the years.

A special note of gratitude must go to the hundreds of people who cooperated in research and development projects with the author over the past four years. This prologue began with a statement about the negative image of the nursing home. This is due in part to a lack of familiarity with nursing homes and the many dedicated people who run them and serve in them. The reason this book can be written is because of the cooperation given unhesitatingly by nursing home administrators and staff personnel. Often, they were the first to recognize a problem, to detail it, and to offer suggestions on how it might be corrected in the future. So many of these professionals and skilled workers suffer under the heavy burden of the image of the nursing home.

This final acknowledgment is perhaps the most important of all. The author is deeply grateful for the help, counsel, and cooperation of the many older Americans who made this work possible and for whom the author hopes the book is in some way helpful in achieving better nursing home environments.

Another important source for any author, researcher, or designer is the writings of others. There are almost too many books, periodicals, and articles—and also important unpublished manuscripts—that have been useful over the years. Many excellent and pivotal writings are not mentioned in this book because the author has decided to limit the references to those pieces worked with directly during research, design development, and writing stages.

Each chapter is followed by a bibliography of selected works that were instrumental as source materials during the preparation of the text. Direct quotations are referenced wherever the quotation appears. Other writings are mentioned without quotes. Owing to the nature of the text, the confluence of many ideas and personal interpretations, and extrapolations and combination with observed phenomena, there is no attempt to provide a comprehensive and detailed literature review.

It is hoped that the nature of the text, its lack of jargon, uncomplicated referencing, and allusions to sources will ensure the widest possible readership and that at least some of the ideas will find their way into the built environment.

Joseph A. Koncelik

CONTENTS

DESIGNING THE
OPEN NURSING HOME

PART I

INTRODUCTION

PROLOGUE

The nursing home is a symbol of the meaning of aging to a great many of the American people, both those over 65 and those many years junior to that age. It is, for the most part, a negative symbol of aging, the last place anyone wants to be. It is largely considered the last place anyone *will* be in their lifetime. The late Seigmund May (1971) referred to the best nursing homes as "gilded cages." The press and other forms of reporting media have thrust scandalous examples of mistreatment and dispair before the collective eyes of the American public, and recent books muckrake the greed of mercenary profiteers in the nursing home business (Mendelson, 1974). There is no escaping the negative image of the nursing home, just as there is no escaping the fact that they are a necessity.

Inevitably, a certain percentage of the aging population must have the advantages of the care that can only be provided effectively and efficiently within an institutional setting. Currently, 5 percent of the elderly or 1 million people live in nursing homes. The rapid growth in the construction of nursing homes in the 1960s is due to a greater consciousness of the needs of older people before and during that period and not because the population in need of nursing care increased all that rapidly. However, since that period, there has been a steady increase in the number of people reaching 65, and more of them are living longer. Thus, greater numbers of people will need some form of assisted living or a supportive environment, even if the percentages remain the same.

Since the nation is faced with expanding and improving the stock of institutional settings as well as other forms of housing for this age range, there should be an attempt to analyze what is known about existing environments and to pass on the knowledge that has accumulated. This text is an attempt to provide some of that knowledge as seen through the eyes and absorbed and transfigured in the mind of one designer. The knowledge of others, who have observed nursing home environments in operation from different vantage points than that of design, should be passed along as well.

Part of the experiences represented in this book is derived from systematic research conducted at two universities. A great many more experiences that have filtered into the writing of the book are informal, impressionistic, and speculative in nature. Only ten institutions are represented in actual research data, but ten times that number have been visited from coast to coast. Experiences gained firsthand have been compared and shared with the experiences of others, so the sum total is a feeling or an attitude about existing environments, what should be done in new buildings, and what changes should be made in the old ones. The book, by the very nature of the subject matter, cannot be comprehensive. More importantly, it is an attempt to share an attitude about people and special environments. It is the author's deeply felt belief that attitudes must change toward the aging population and toward nursing homes before any truly meaningful change will come about.

Design is in the end only a reflection of attitudes. Designers are not in the position to change attitudes, as so many have so painfully learned over time. When a meaningful change of direction in design seems feasible to a designer, the designer must wait until attitudes permit the change in design process. The waiting has become too painful with regard to nursing home design; perhaps, then, this book is as much an expression of frustration as well as specification of needs.

Supporting the nursing home concept is not an argument in support of no other form of environment for the aging population. To be sure, a variety of levels of care should be provided. Living units that support and maintain independence should be provided. Homes and apartments not specifically designated as elderly living units should also be designed, extending the view of who inhabits to include the elderly. All these things should be part of a general concern of meeting the needs of the total elderly population.

Perhaps one of the most important ways in which the needs of the elderly population can be met is to include them as common denominators for all design activities. Currently, designers use an extremely abstract model of the human being as a starting point for the design of all products, general interiors, and architecture. Holding up the model of an elderly person as a measure against which these designs are made accountable would reveal many potential changes and improvements that could be made, most with relative ease. This point of departure is beginning to be taken seriously by some industrial

designers as well as architects and interior designers. Once industry realizes that the changes might mean expanding product sales, as well as making objects and spaces more useful for everyone, there may well be sweeping changes in the consumer products and architectural hardware everyone has struggled with for so long.

To return to the subject of this book, there is no avoiding the necessity and efficacy of the nursing home. However, regardless of official designations, they are all "closed" systems of care. There are many ways to enter, but almost no ways to get out of the system once the aging patient-resident has become a part of that system.

The "open" system of care or support is ideally a system that has at least as many apertures for getting out of the system as there are for getting in. This concept presupposes the wild idea that everyone not only wants to leave this level of intensive medical-supportive atmosphere but that they *will* leave it alive. This is a wild idea because not everyone will; but the attitude must be there in spite of the statistical realities. When attitudes change, so do the statistics.

Whether official designations label institutions as extended care facilities, skilled nursing homes, convalescent homes, county infirmary, and so on, they are all providing constant nursing care. It has been shown in several studies and very well described in an article by J. Ronald D. Bayne (1971) in the *Gerontologist* that the intensive nature and overall atmosphere created are conducive to dependency on the health care delivery system for continuing support. The harder concept to make work is one whereby the health care system does not predominate in the environment. This major shift in emphasis within these settings is the pivotal idea for all other changes, which eventually manifest in an entirely different concept of physical environment.

Openness in the general scheme of nursing home care also necessitates an end to the antiquated notion that effective delivery of services to the community—specifically to elderly individuals living independently—would eliminate the need for institutional settings housing confined and constrained aging people. First, there are no comprehensive data that show the superiority or economic cost effectiveness of either delivery system over the other. Second, the nursing home has been used frequently as a base of operations for community, areawide delivery of services. Third, no nursing home should be used to house aging people who are not in need of health care on a continual monitored basis.

Openness in the concept of nursing home care means utilization of all services ordinarily provided in the nursing home by the community. Likewise, it means incorporation of the community into the concept of the nursing home operation. There are a wide variety of programmatic opportunities that are viable services and also become the much needed "apertures" for exit from the health care environment. These include the delivery of hot meals to indigent elderly people, day care programs for elderly, incorporation of foster grandparent programs, outpatient programs, sheltered workshop programs for those who reside in the institutions, open meals programs within the setting, activity and educational programs beyond occupational therapy for both the residents and nonresidents of the nursing home, and many more opportunities. It should be obvious that, if an attitude exists whereby even one open program is incorporated, many more are possible and will probably follow.

An open nursing home would also include aging residents on boards of directors and in consultative capacities. These characteristics might be harder to accept, but attempts should be made to achieve their acceptance.

For the purposes of this document, it is desirable to disregard the regulatory structures that abound concerning the nursing home. The one pervasive problem with codes is that they are derived from hospital models—just reduced in the concept of intensity of care. To provide a sense of openness in a conceptualization of nursing homes, it is necessary to address the inhabitants as something more than patients. The model of the hospital, then, does not provide the proper perspective for an effective visualization or conceptualization of the physical setting end product.

Openness at the onset of this discussion also precludes entanglements with the complexities of a health care financing mechanism, such as Medicare

or any other financial support structure. America is progressing toward a goal of national health care in some form or other. This many-headed hydra has not evolved to its final form. Hopefully, national health planning will mean integration of various programs in health care and building. Why predicate a model for nursing home care or physical plant development on programs that literally convulse with change every year of their existence? It is better to reach beyond current restrictions that are transitory and suggest ideas less subject to obsolescence. In this spirit, it is possible to conceptualize a new, responsive, flexible, and compassionate concept of care, as well as a concept of design echoing these ideas.

The essential consideration for openness in the institutional setting is an intent to maximize independence and to minimize or withdraw support to the lowest possible level. This is easier written about than instituted. The designers and planners of institutional space must constantly exercise diligence in finding ways to make their designs serve these ends.

One essential characteristic of the open approach is to predicate design on the needs of the aging who reside in these structures and not on the needs of the staff. Obviously, the needs of both groups must be met because they are users of the same space. However, health care is dispensed, it is given, and this mandates a receiver; it implies authority and submissiveness. It has been shown in the work of M. Powell Lawton (1970a, 1970b, 1975) that the less submissive patients in a nursing home setting and elderly occupants of public housing often fare better than their more docile cohorts. There is hope on this front, to be sure; those who reach old age currently are far less docile and far more demanding, as well as being better educated and more familiar with mobility and the American life style of change.

There is a long history of books, articles, and reports generated over the past 40 years dealing with the subject matter found in this document. The sources upon which an experience was built to make this book possible would be too numerous to mention in totality. It is therefore more appropriate to attempt to capture the trends that were generated over the years to show why the state of the art is what it is and where gaps in present knowledge lie.

There is no definitive history of the nursing home on a national scale, but William C. Thomas's *Nursing Homes and Public Policy in New York State* provides excellent background and insights into the shifts in emphasis in care of the elderly over the years. Unfortunately, both the public and those professionals concerned about care of the elderly tend to forget the past and its bitter lessons. This book shows that the argument over home health care versus institutional care has been taking place for almost 100 years. From time to time, victory in the shape of public policy has shifted from one side of this argument to the other. Scandals have abounded in this area of health care and show no sign of dissipating.

Real concern in the form of research investigations, governmental inquiry, and professional development for geriatric specialties took root and began rapid growth in the 1950s. In this period, several pieces of literature were written that could be labeled "specifications." Glenn Beyer (1954) and Alex Kira (1960) developed research and then documentation they called "requirements." Wilma Donahue's (1966) contribution to a greater understanding of the relationship of self-reliance to environment can also be seen as part of this trend. There are others.

In the late 1950s and through to the mid-1960s, for about a decade, there was an incredible push to construct a large variety of housing and institutional settings for the elderly. At that time there seemed to be a confluence of available resources, demand, professional concern, and determination to build. In a survey of the literature of this period, Koncelik and Edelsberg (1972) found that determination to build superseded the knowledge of what to build. Ollie Randall, the noted gerontologist, said it best when she reflected a few years ago, "We built in ignorance, but we had to build." Unfortunately, this country is left with the legacy of mistakes and ignorance in brick and mortar—difficult to live with (Figure 1), but equally difficult to find the motivation to change.

During the same period of time, architects and planners documented the construction process. Mathiasen et al. (1959), Musson and Hevsinkveld (1963), Weiss, and others wrote prolifically on this subject. Noakes stated in 1959 that the specification for building was a "vague outline." Joseph Weiss wrote later in 1969 that information about the "ecology of aging" and "proxemics," a word coined by anthropologist Hall (1969) to signify the interrelationship of man to object in a psychophysical sense, was influencing designers and the design process, but the information was inconclusive. The sad truth is the boom in institutional building took place without a coherent body of knowledge having been assembled on these and other subjects within the framework of the human factors of aging.

There may have been no choice. The nation was faced with a growing population of aging people living in environments where they were inadequately cared for. They were scattered about in old converted dwellings or inappropriate structures that were dangerous, unsanitary, and overcrowded. New York State records show that the average population in institutional settings before the boom in construction was four people. Ten years later the average was 26. In another 10 years, the average nationally may well be above 100 people per institutional setting. It is not uncommon today to find campus-type facilities with multiple levels of care having as many as 900 or more residents. In a general sense and to a large degree, the institutional setting for the aged infirm has greatly inproved along with the care, but the environments are tremendously different and have generated an unusual model concept.

In the rush to improve the more glaring faults of institutional care, those things which were less tangible—sense of being, dignity, socialization, and occupation—were trampled and left undeveloped or given short shrift in the newer settings. The clinical atmosphere of most nursing homes today is overpowering even to the visitor. The quietude, sterility, and sameness from area to area are oppressive. Also, though the psychological and social atmospheres were not tangibles when construction was at its height, they are more tangible in very sizable bodies of information today. Ironically, this information has largely been gathered from the very buildings, the institutions built during the late 1950s and 1960s, constructed in hasty ignorance in the first place.

It is not feasible to demolish what has been built and not possible to turn back the clock. Changes can be made to existing structures that will help to ameli-

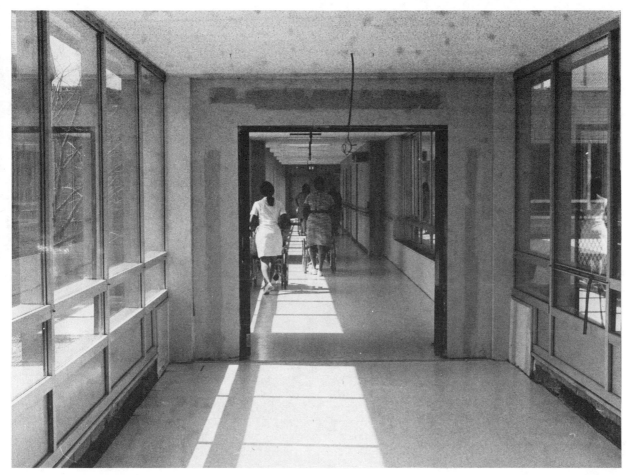

FIGURE 1
A barrier to access, the long corridor. (Photo: David O. Watkins.)

orate some of the problems created. New construction will be going on into the foreseeable future. There will not be the great boom of construction of the 1950s and 1960s; but there will be steady new development and a great deal of refurbishing and conversion. Interiors are largely modifiable and furnishings must be replaced periodically. The inexorable act of wear will dictate change, and this change should be studied, monitored, and accomplished on a progressive basis in the large majority of existing buildings.

As the boom in construction has curtailed, the relationship of man and environment, especially the psychological and social environment, has become of greater interest to many researchers. In fact, this area has received a great deal of attention in the last five years. The behavioral context, however, is only part of a larger concern over human factors. This area of study embraces the physiological aspects of environmental design as well. Only when the marriage of these elements of the human condition with respect to environment is accomplished will a truly effective approach to designing any environment for any population be realized.

At present, environmental studies emphasize mainly the psychological and sociological aspects of the impact of physical settings on users. The traditional human factors or human engineering approach is to catalogue physiological attributes of the human being and allow designers to project the use of these data. Still another field measures "psychophysical" responses to environmental stimuli.

These separate areas of study, largely constrained owing to monodisciplinary generation, must be amalgamated if environmental studies, environmental analysis, man–environment interfaces, and the like, are to become useful. Only with an approach in which various factors are weighed, evaluated, and systematically ordered can there be a comprehensive and balanced approach to designing environments for any age group or range.

At the moment, it is the hapless designer who accepts the responsibility for integrating or disregarding the information on environmental impact upon the user. Although the designer is not in a position to set initial specifications for designs, the ultimate responsibility for the judgments necessary to formulate designs is the designer's. If a balanced approach is to be achieved, the design process must be opened up to include other disciplines willing to share the responsibilities. This is hard to achieve because designing is a risk. Likewise, an unfortunate aspect of the development of information in environmental subject areas is that they are treated exclusively within professional bounds. The point of social and psychological data on environment, and especially information in these areas, is that they should lead to better environments. To do this, the information must be interpretable by others who build, program, and deliver care. At present, much information which could be used or applied is too riddled with jargon and unidisciplinary orientated to be of use in the design process. This problem could be ameliorated by having designers learn research techniques and participate in data collection.

Robert Sommer (1969, 1972) is a leading behavioral scientist concerned with environments and the design of settings for behaviors. His experience, described in his book, *Design Awareness*, demonstrates the need for multidisciplinary and interdisciplinary study of environment and design of environments. The designer must enter the information generation process in order to ensure that usable and interpretable data are collected and documented. The human factors specialist must accept partial responsibility for the generation of designs to ensure the highest possible level of human satisfaction. To be sure, the strategies and techniques are available for this process to be undertaken.

Gerontology, an umbrella that covers many disciplines working with the aging and on problems of aging, is a field in which a significant step has been taken toward developing relationships on multidisciplinary and interdisciplinary bases. One important factor that has compelled more of this type of professional relationships is the degree to which the elderly are sensitive to their surroundings. Interest in environments for the aging is keen because they are very sensitive to changes in their surroundings as well as to stability in their surroundings. The largest portion, fully 80 percent of the elderly (over 65), have a chronic physical problem. This in large measure is the key element in this strong relationship between the aging individual and his environment. As chronic problems turn to more serious health problems and incapacities, this relationship turns to dependency. At this point, literally every element of the environment has a significance. The absence of certain qualities may have even more significance.

In the broad field of gerontology, many researchers, designers, and other professionals have recorded relationships between environment and the aging. An important work in this area is the book by Carson and Pastalan, *Spatial Behavior of Older People*. M. Powell Lawton has written prolifically in this same area and others connected with aging. The aforementioned Robert Sommer's *Personal Space* and *Design Awareness* are important references for those concerned about the environment, both for the aging population and other generations.

In the field of gerontology and in the study and design of nursing homes, there is a lesson to be learned by designers and researchers who are not involved with the problems of aging people. The interchange between professions, the lack of concern for disciplinary boundaries, has promulgated some of the most interesting work in the whole arena of man-environment relationships. It is safe to say that there is really no place for those who are interested in exclusivity in the field of gerontology. The concern of virtually everyone involved with the aging and the aging process is helping to solve problems associated with age. If this attitude could be accepted by a larger group or by all those involved with the study and creation of environments, there would be many, many more significant improvements for everyone.

REFERENCES

Bayne, J. Ronald D. "Environmental Modification for the Older Person." *The Gerontologist*, 11, no. 4 (1971), pt. I.

Beattie, Walter M. "The Design of Supportive Environments for the Life Span." *The Gerontologist*, 10, no. 3 (1970).

Beyer, Glenn H. *The Cornell Kitchen: Product Design Through Research*. Ithaca, N.Y.: Cornell University, 1954.

——, and Sylvia Wahl. *Economic Aspects of Housing for the Aged*. Ithaca, N.Y.: Cornell Research Program on Housing for the Aged, 1961.

——, and Sylvia Wahl. *The Elderly and Their Housing*. Ithaca, N.Y.: Cornell University Experiment Station, 1963.

——, and Margaret W. Wood. *Living and Activity Patterns of the Aged*. Ithaca, N.Y.: Cornell Center for Housing and Environmental Studies, 1963.

Carson, Donald H., and Leon D. Pastalan. *Spatial Behavior of Older People*. Ann Arbor, Mich.: Institute of Gerontology, University of Michigan, 1970.

Donahue, Wilma. "Impact of Living Arrangements on Ego Development in the Elderly," in *Patterns of Living and Housing Middle Aged and Older People*. U.S. Public Health Service, Department of Health, Education, and Welfare, Rockville, Md., 1966, pub. no. 1496.

Hall, Edward T. *The Hidden Dimension*. Garden City, N.Y.: Doubleday & Company, Inc., 1969.

Kira, Alexander. *The Bathroom: Criteria for Design*. Ithaca, N.Y.: Cornell University Center for Housing and Environmental Studies, 1966.

——. "Housing Needs of the Aged." *Rehabilitation Literature* (National Society for Crippled Children and Adults), 21, no. 12 (1960), pp. 370-377, 384.

——, et al. *Housing Requirements of the Aged: A Study of Design Criteria*. Albany, N.Y.: New York State Division of Housing, 1958.

Lawton, M. Powell. "Ecology and Aging." In *Spatial Behavior of Older People*, L. D. Pastalan and D. H. Carson (eds.). Ann Arbor, Mich.: Institute of Gerontology, University of Michigan, 1970a, pp. 40-67.

——. "Planner's Notebook: Planning Environments for Older People." *AIP Journal*, 36, no. 2 (1970b).

——. *Planning and Managing Housing for the Elderly*. New York: John Wiley & Sons, Inc., 1975.

Mathiasen, Genava, Edward Noakes, et al. *Planning Homes for the Aged*. New York: McGraw-Hill, Inc., 1959.

May, Seigmund H. "An Environment for the Aging." In *Environments for the Aging: Selected Talks in Seminar*, J. A. Koncelik (Ed.). Mimeographed. Ithaca, N.Y.: College of Human Ecology, Cornell University, 1971.

Mead, G. H. *Mind, Self, and Society: From the Standpoint of a Social Behaviorist*. Chicago: University of Chicago, 1934.

Mendelson, Mary A. *Tender Loving Greed*. New York: Random House, Inc., 1974.

Musson, Noverre, and Helen Hevsinkveld. *Buildings for the Elderly*. New York: Van Nostrand Reinhold Company, 1963.

Neugarten, Bernice. "The Awareness of Middle Age." In *Middle Age and Aging*, B. Neugarten (ed.). Chicago: University of Chicago Press, 1968, pp. 93-98.

Pirsig, Robert. *Zen and the Art of Motorcycle Maintenance*. New York: William Morrow & Company, Inc., 1974.

Sommer, Robert. *Personal Space*. Englewood Cliffs, N.J.: Prentice-Hall, Inc., 1969.

——. *Design Awareness*. New York: Holt, Rinehart and Winston, Inc., 1972.

Thomas, William C. *Nursing Homes and Public Policy in New York State*. Ithaca, N.Y.: Cornell University Press, 1971.

Weiss, Joseph D. *Better Buildings for the Aged*. New York: Hopkinson and Blake, 1969.

**Publications from Cornell Research Projects
(as of June 1973)**

Koncelik, Joseph A. "Design to Meet Patient Needs and Enhance Longevity of the Long Term Care Facility." *Empire State Architect*, 32, no. 1 (1972).

——. "Environmental Effects upon the Institutionalized Aging and Aging People Affecting Their Environment." *The Designer*, 16, no. 180 (1972).

——. "The Future of Aging in America." *Human Ecology Forum*, 1, no. 3 (1971).

——, and Susan Edelsberg. *Considerate Design and the Aging*. Council of Planning Librarians Exchange Bibliographies, no. 253 (Jan. 1972).

——, and Edward Ostrander. "Architectural Barriers and the Voiceless Consumer." *Human Ecology Forum*, 2, no. 2 (1971).

——, and Lorraine H. Snyder. "The Role of Design in Behavior Manipulation Within Long Term Care Facilities." *Nursing Homes*, 20, no. 12 (1971).

Snyder, Lorraine H. "A Case in Point: The Geriatric Wheelchair." *Human Ecology Forum*, 3, no. 2 (1972).

——. *The Environmental Challenge and the Aging Individual*. Council of Planning Librarians Exchange Bibliographies, no. 254 (Jan. 1972).

——, Edward Ostrander, and Joseph Koncelik. *The New Nursing Home*. Conference Proceedings, College of Human Ecology, Cornell University, Ithaca, N.Y. (June 1973).

Steidl, Rose E., and Linda Nelson. *The Ergonomics of Environmental Design and Activity Management for the Aging*. Council of Planning Librarians Exchange Bibliographies, no. 255 (Jan. 1972).

PART **II**

BACKGROUND
ON THE POPULATION

PHYSIOLOGICAL ASPECTS OF AGING AS DESIGN DETERMINANTS

Virtually all fields of design treat subject matter in the area of human factors with some degree of respect. Not all design decisions are based on information about user characteristics, but it is a basis for the great majority of design decisions. The difficulty is that the greatest volume of human factors information is abstracted to such a degree as to preclude characteristics of the aging population. In essence, the abstract "model" human man–woman used as a predictive tool in the design process is quite young, vigorous, and supple. Compared with the large number of aging people—even those over 50—this model is godlike. In other words, the human body is characterized in information most designers use as existing in a static state: a kind of suspended youth in maturity, fully developed and eternally young.

There is extensive written material on the physiology of aging, but none recorded in the kind of usable form designers rely upon. An image must be created to make the information usable. This chapter is a synthesis of some of the more important pieces of information about the physiological aspects of the aging process. Technical jargon and medical terminology have been purposely reduced or their use avoided; the emphasis is on expanding traditional no-

tions about human factors to include information about the aging.

There are artificial determinants of age that society finds expedient. The arbitrary cutoff of 65 as a chronological measure of ability is not very reliable in measuring true capability. Physiological appearance is a deception. Gray hair and wrinkles may show that one person has been around longer than another, but it will not act as an accurate predictor of capability. Generally, those reaching retirement age are reaching it in better condition than in the past. The problem is that health is not a constant which suddenly evaporates at the onset of death. Everyone tends to change or "develop" both physiologically and in other ways throughout the life span and especially in advanced years.

Although not visual and less institutional than retirement, real aging is measured by the loss of reserve or the decline in the body's ability to maintain homeostasis. Homeostasis refers to the equilibrium of interactions among organs, glands, muscles, bone, and tissue in the human system. At rest, this system is said to be homeostatic. When the body works or exerts energy, muscle tissue, the lungs, and other parts of the body require more oxygen and nutrients. The body attempts to furnish these requirements to establish or reestablish equilibrium. In youth, there is strength, suppleness, and expansive development; reserve is high. With advancing age, there is loss of strength, a lessening of the supply of oxygen and nutrients through the respiration and circulation systems so that the body has either a harder job or, in some cases, an impossible task in reestablishing homeostasis. This is indeed an oversimplification of the concept, but it illustrates a key difference between youthful physiology and that of the aging. There is less tolerance of physical stress.

Two other concepts must be shared at this point. First, not all facets of the aging process are losses. There are gains, especially in terms of continuing development up to a point. A greater effort should be mounted to establish more data on adult development. Most developmental work has been done using children as subjects. This stems from a natural bias, that because children grow they develop. This bias maintains that the human organism levels off in development and then declines, losing capabilities with age. This is in many ways an untrue and unfair assumption. It was shown many years ago that, although older adults accept information at a slower rate than do children and young adults, their retention and comprehension is just as high, if not higher in some cases, than the young. There may be other capacities that have an upward or increasing development with age; but more intensive study in the area of adult development must be done to establish this information.

A second important factor in the human organism's aging process is the effect of cultural norms and dictates. Americans have reacted to industrialization and material acquisition by becoming sedentary and developing poor nutritional habits. Lack of exercise, use of stimulants and depressants, poor diet, smoking and drinking in excess hasten age in the physiological sense on top of leading to heart disease, cancer, and respiratory and circulatory problems. It is possible that regular exercise and careful diet control could prolong reserve just as lack of control hastens its demise.

The inertia of the social and cultural environment is such that there is little hope of making great inroads into the socialization process which leads the majority of the population toward a sedentary life. To accept the definition of aging as a loss of physiological reserve means that many others who are below the age of 65 are indeed among those who must be classified as in the ranks of the aged. Likewise, many who are over the age of 65 do not classify as aged.

The subject of death is usually connected with the subject of aging. However, death is not necessarily a result of aging or the process of reserve loss. The human organism is capable of delivering adequate or more than adequate performance even with substantial loss of reserve capacity. Death is being studied from many standpoints. The Kubler–Ross (1969) studies with terminal patients are an important contribution to the understanding of the phenomenon. Recently, studies of transfers from one setting to another among the aging infirm show that the anticipated move may provide a threat to an aging person who is in need of stability. Recent research in this area shows that one of the most reliable predictors of death among the elderly who have been transferred from one setting to another may be the loss of desire to penetrate the social and physical environment. The number of times a person needs to go beyond his or her boundaries—or have someone penetrate theirs—in order to remain alive can be fixed. These numbers of penetrations become the most accurate predictor of death among the aging who have been transferred from one setting to another (Pastalan, 1974).

Autopsies have revealed other interesting aspects about death. Often someone who has endured a long life has done so with many pathological conditions, any one of which might have been the cause of death at any time. Younger adults have died suddenly from the first pathological condition that afflicted them.

There seems to be a strong connection between the will to live and the maintenance of life itself. This connection has been a suspicion for many years and is now being confirmed with study on an empirical basis.

Designers of nursing homes and those concerned about the spaces and objects surrounding the aging are almost totally concerned with the human organism in the normal state and not with death. The crucial question is how does the environment impede or facilitate the life of the aging who reside in any given environment? M. Powell Lawton (1970) has professed that the more a person loses capabilities to negotiate environments the more that person becomes dependent on the environment for support. This concept has been referred to by Lawton as the "environmental docility hypothesis." As strength fails and as the sensory organs incur deprivations, the individual experiencing these losses reaches out to both the general social environment and the physical environment in order to continue functioning.

The nursing home is obviously then a supportive or "prosthetic" environment. As aging people decline in health, and yet desire to continue to function, the environment must be so designed to accommodate whatever level of functioning the aging and infirm person is capable of. These "users" of the environment are *special users:* residents who need supportive health care in an enriched environment.

HOMEOSTASIS

Homeostasis is the state of equilibrium or balance of all the functions of the body. The human organism interacts with its environment to sustain itself, and through breathing, eating, eliminating wastes, and repairing damaged tissue regulates itself to achieve equilibrium (Reichenbach and Mathers, 1959). The involuntary nervous system maintains equilibrium by regulating heart rate, blood pressure, body temperature, and so on. When the body is placed under physiological stress, there are changes in functions to accommodate the demands of the muscles, tissue, organs, and other parts of the body. A young adult may possess several times the capacity to produce blood, pump it, and work hard for durations of time than he or she needs when in a state of equilibrium. This *reserve* capacity is essential in bringing the bodily functions back to a normal steady state.

Sometime after 30 years, there begins a steady decline in the reserve capacity of the body. Actual inception of declines in reserve vary widely among people. However, there are steady losses of strength, ability to produce and pump blood, and other declines in capability. As time goes on, there are hearing losses (Birren, 1964), some of which are not correctable

prosthetically, sight impairments, and generally greater susceptibility to illness, accidents, and exposure.

An elderly person in seemingly good health may not have any reserve capacity at all. An infirm elderly person could potentially lack homeostasis even at rest so that his or her body is never in a state of balance. When health declines, the effects may be unpredictable. Organs that have not been affected by an illness are affected because of the loss of reserve and inability to receive the necessary blood supply or other sustaining nutrients or repairs.

While cellular levels remain approximately the same, there is an undeniable loss of performance at the organic level. With this decrease is a concurrent reduction in overall body metabolism and resistance to disease, a stage referred to as "senescence" or senile stage (Gerard, 1959).

PHYSIOLOGICAL SYSTEM DYSFUNCTION AFFECTING HOMEOSTASIS

The mechanisms affecting homeostasis that regulate and integrate the human organism are classified as endocrine, autonomic (sympathetic and parasympathetic nervous system regulation), and circulatory. With age there is a decline in their speed of action and potency (Shock, 1952; Comfort, 1956; Gerard, 1959). According to investigators of the physiological aspects of aging, the human organism ultimately will die of old age owing to a lack of ability to self-regulate. The signals being given and received in the body are no longer coordinated or sequential. Behavioral and social failures can be attributed to failures of the central nervous system (Gerard, 1959).

Alterations in physiological controls make death more highly probable. The malfunctioning of the homeostatic mechanism may explain why old people are less resistant to disease, why they incur less efficient or disturbed functioning of major organs, nervous system, the endocrines, and so on, under stress or disease. It may also explain why they die in greater numbers than other segments of the population.

Physiological detriments and general performance losses can be viewed as a negative development in aging. However, it is important to keep in mind that these phenomena are progressive, subtle, and slow in most cases. Realization of the aging process is often not possible unless the organism is placed in a situation of stress or with the inception of illness. So Kuhlen (1959) points out, *adjustment* over time is central to the adaptability of the organism. Aging is a dynamic process allowing people to live up to potential and to change psychologically with physiological change.

External or internal stimulation to the aging organism with conditions of dysfunction will cause a reaction in the organism, which reflects an imbalance and heightened susceptibility. Older people are less able to adapt to extremes in temperature, either high or low. The band of tolerance becomes narrower with age. Possible reasons for this lessened adaptability are lessened heat production (metabolism), impairment of heat loss through the skin, lessened musculature and capacity of the muscles, and altered response of tissue to thyroid hormones. More important is the reaction to physical work in a state of increasing dysfunction.

One of the important areas of study of work under stress is the investigation of work in high and low temperatures (Kleemeier, 1959; Krag and Kountz, 1950, 1952; Horvath et al., 1955). Readjustment of the heart rate and breathing rate to normal takes longer for older adults than for young people. Likewise, readjustment after stress in high temperatures takes longer for older people. The research on reaction to cold temperatures is inconclusive with some saying the older adult is less efficient in preventing heat loss, while others (Horvath et al., 1955) state that the elderly seem less susceptible to cold. It is likely that extremes of temperature for physiological work–stop are not good. The research in this area, however, is inconclusive.

Old people die in greater numbers than the rest of the population. This seems overly obvious to generations born in the latter half of this century. However, this was not always the case. Children had the highest rate of mortality up until recently in the majority of cultures; they still do in a great number. The average life expectancy has shown a dramatic increase largely because childhood diseases have been eliminated. In truth, although we assume that science and technology have added years to our lives, only four years of additional life have been added since the turn of the century. There is a great interest in extending life today. Basic research findings make the argument that the potential of the human organism is 150 to 200 years. However, getting the human body to sustain life that long is an enormous cultural, social, and ideological problem. The scientific advances being made in preventing and curing cardiac disease and cancer really means that many more people will be making it into their 60's, 70's, and 80's rather than extending life beyond the commonly accepted averages. It also means that *many more people will require supportive environments as their physical conditions will be impaired.*

Closer examination is warranted of the organs and other systems that make up the complex interrelationships of the human body. Six divisions for further study are the endocrines, the nervous system, cellular structures, musculoskeletal system, the major organs, and the sensory channels.

THE AGING ENDOCRINE SYSTEM

The biological aspects of aging are not readily classified as simply time related phenomena. Each organism is a complex mixture of interrelated genetic and environmental factors.

Certain biological functions show a downward trend in capacity with aging. These include changes in the endocrine system. Changes take place regardless of whether or not the aging person has had a disease. In later life, it can be difficult to separate or distinguish between the actual health status of an aged person and whether or not they have a disease. However, it should be noted that physiologists and medical professionals do not feel that all changes in the endocrine system are degenerative.

The endocrine system, or glandular system, is generally reduced in effectiveness, secretive capacity, and interaction of hormones. There is a general decrease in adrenal activity, decreases in basal metabolism, and changes in the reproductive organs. Under stress, parallel to other bodily functions under stress, there is an exaggerated decrease in the effectiveness and interaction of hormones. The decrease in adrenal activity hampers adaptation to physical stress. The processing capacity of the body to handle sugars decreases with age because there are fewer cells to do the processing. The most obvious change in the glandular system is the change in the gonadal glands. Women cease menstruating at some point in the middle years. In men, there is a decrease in the production of spermatozoa, but relatively little decrease in male hormones.

Masters and Johnson (1966) have done a more comprehensive study of geriatric sexual response and the changes in sexuality related to aging. Their findings indicate that, although there are progressive atrophic changes in organ function, sexual relations may be enjoyed well into the eightieth year—providing there has been a healthy attitude toward sexuality in the first place and regular, nonepisodic sexual activity in the second. One of the greatest problems for women is the lack of a partner in advanced years, while men are subject to societal stresses that curtail their desire for sexual activity. Overeating, and especially excessive ingestion of alcohol, are seen as detriments to long-term sexual fulfillment as well.

The work in the field of sexual response brings into focus the unavoidable physiological as well as social fact that women outlive men, and that the human needs upon which nursing home design is predicated are largely the needs of women. Also, this society's concepts about sexual activity and morality in general are changing and the role of the woman is changing. It is likely that the future nursing home facility may have to provide for human needs, such as privacy for sexual activity, on a larger basis than in the past. The Victorian attitudes that predominate among today's elderly will be a thing of the past by the turn of the century. There is probably little hope that men will live longer and in greater numbers in advanced years, but certainly the women who reach old age will not be docile, recessive, and dependent creatures as they have been.

There have been many books related to the changing role of women, but the seminal work is Simone De Beauvoir's *The Second Sex*. It is especially important to refer to in the context of aging because De Beauvoir writes so beautifully and so sensibly about the role of women throughout the life span and not as an abstracted, alienated, and political creature. The "physi-ologic" and "psychophysical" woman is changing—becoming more conscious of her real place and, in later years, her predominance.

The social and cultural norms affecting all people dictate a lessening of sexual activity as age increases. It would seem that one of the greatest and most falsely determined social taboos in Western culture is the taboo on sexual activity for the aging. This society seems ready to accept the onset of sexual activity at earlier ages, perhaps with onerous social consequences; but it is difficult for most younger adults to accept that their grandfathers and grandmothers are engaging in something that has been a part of their lives for decades.

THE NERVOUS SYSTEM AND THE BRAIN

The main detrimental occurrence of significance in the neurological system is cellular degeneration as age progresses. Cell loss with advanced years can account for a drop of 25 to 44 percent in brain weight. This cellular loss is reflected in slowing of reaction time and response. Blood flow to the brain decreases by as much as 20 percent. However, this decrease is not as great as the decreases in other parts of the body, because the body is shunting blood from other areas to the brain to preserve its critical function.

The brain, however, contains many more millions of cells than the human organism will ever use. Though reaction time and response are slowed, the intellectual process overall remains largely intact. Research conducted over many years has shown that, in learning situations where the pace is fast, elderly people will have a hard time keeping up and comprehending. If learning time is allowed to extend or the pace is slowed, elderly people learn as well as any other age group. Erroneous conclusions have been drawn about the ability to learn and general intellectual capacity by referring to cross-sectional studies of intelligence. These data show differences in intelligence levels between generations. However, they have often been used to illustrate decline with age, and this has not been proved by these studies. Longitudinal studies have been done to some degree. They are harder to carry out because they require years of follow up and a maintenance of techniques and, ideally, research teams. When they have been conducted, they show little or no decrease in learning capacity or potential. This information is yet inconclusive, and it is linked clearly to what should be an expanded effort in adult development. It is safe to say that comparisons of 18-year-old students and 75-year-old adults who have not had the same educational intensity in their lives are unwise and unfair.

It should be noted that longitudinal studies have shown a great loss in intellectual capability just two years before death. It is possible that monitoring the activity, both social and intellectual, may provide clues about the onset of death.

There is cell loss throughout the central nervous system, which also accounts for a slowing of response and reaction. As a result of this general depreciation, forms of organic dementia may occurr. There may be a rigidity of reaction and hence a need for stability or constancy; new places or conditions may precipitate confusion; there may be many overt reactions to failing memory—compulsiveness, a need for repitition, and the like.

Problems related to organic dementia include an inability to discriminate between sounds or a tendency to misinterpret them. Background noises can be confused with the human voice. Approxia, a motor disorder of the neurological system resulting from generalized cell loss, is a loss of the concept of movement, as if a person has forgotten how to walk. Once underway, movement is possible until the person stops; then remembering how to start is difficult. An aged person with this disorder may lean backward or forward, depending on which side of the brain is affected, and fall at times.

The elderly may also suffer peripheral neuropathesis, which is a loss of reflexes and area sensation. This disorder can be caused nutritionally through exposure to toxicity or through metabolic disorders such as diabetes.

There are spinal syndromes such as compression of the spinal vasculature, an extremely painful disorder. Disc degeneration and other disorders threaten the spinal cord and the central nervous system.

Common cranial disorders include Paget's disease, which includes symptoms of paralysis, palsy, and progressive deafness. Trigeminal neuralgia causes severe head pains, and temporal arthritis causes pain in the scalp and face.

THE AGING MUSCULOSKELETAL SYSTEM

Many researchers feel that the deterioration and reduction of oxygen consumption is directly related to the aging of the muscles and skeleton. Aging of these two interrelated components of the body is also related to alterations in metabolism. As loss of high-oxygen-producing cell mass progresses, there is increased vulnerability to disease and loss of homeostatic balance.

Peak muscle strength occurs between 20 and 30 years and declines progressively thereafter. Muscle strength decreases to approximately 55 percent of what it had been at 30 sometime in the 70's. However, exercise is extremely important in maintaining fitness and reserve in later years. Walking, or exercising the leg muscles, improves the strength of the cardiac muscle and improves circulation. Constancy of an exercise program can reduce the severity of artereosclerotic lesions and incidence of thrombosis and embolism. Active leg contraction, walking or jogging, yields 30 percent or more of the power required to sustain movement of blood, thus actually reducing work stress on the heart.

There are five ways that muscle fiber changes:

1. Decrease in the number of fibers.
2. Decrease in fiber bulk.
3. Decreases due to atrophy of other organs.
4. Conspicuous or visible changes, such as thinning of the hands or flabbiness of the arms.
5. Progressive muscular atrophy, recognized as severe weakness.

Significant changes in posture take place with aging. The head and neck are extended farther forward than in youth, the spine becomes curved, the upper limbs bent at the elbows and wrists, and the hips and knees flexed. These manifestations are due to changes in the vestibular column in discs, changes in ligaments and joints, shrinkage of tendons and muscles, and degeneration in the central nervous system. There is also progressive muscular rigidity.

Walking patterns change. Studies such as those of

Murray et al. (1969) show gait changes due to normal change and disease. In general, the gait can be described subjectively as guarded and reserved. There are shorter and broader strides to provide greater stability.

Tremor is significant in the elderly. It will appear with tiredness or early after waking. It reduces the ability to make discriminant small motor maneuvers or control adjustments, such as dialing a telephone.

Neuromuscular disorders occurring with age result in weakness, muscular wasting, stiffness, and spasms. Spinal cord tremors result in weakness and abnormal movements of the body.

The skeletal system is made vulnerable to accident and trauma, which usually results in greater damage because of lessening resiliency. Common occurrences after falls and other accidents are fractures of the pelvis, femur, and spine. This increased vulnerability is brought on by decreased homeostatic efficiency and vital capacity. Bone density is lower in later life.

Osteoporosis is found with increasing frequency in old age. It is a metabolic disorder of the body characterized by an abnormal porousness of the bones due to enlarged bone canals. Fully 10 percent of the population over 50, or 10 million people, have varying degrees of osteoporosis. Comparatively, Paget's disease is found in 4 percent of the general population. Osteoporosis results in thickened bones, especially the skull, and deformities of the humerus, femur, and tibia.

The general health and performance of the bones, joints, muscles, cartilege, and skin depend largely on a substance called collogen. This is a gelatinous mass found in connective tissue, and it contributes about 40 percent of the body protein needed in these areas. It may influence recovery after stress, such as after surgery, and assist in the healing process. Surgery becomes a more difficult proposition in old age. Pathologic conditions and health in general can be affected by surgery in unpredictable ways. Homeostasis is upset generally during and after surgery. In the case where the patient is aged, homeostasis and reserve are not necessarily normal to begin with.

In research tracing the repair and recovery from hip fractures in a small sample of patients, 15 other pathologies were significant in these patients' case histories. Some of these conditions included artereosclerosis, cataract, diabetes, emphysema, arthritis, and Parkinsonism. Several of the patients had more than one disease.

Arthritis is common among the aging. Practically every person alive will have arthritis to some degree in some form before death. Statistics vary on the pervasiveness of arthritis in the American population, but it must be considered one of the most prominent disabling conditions, if not the most disabling condition afflicting man. The Arthritis Foundation counts 17 million people afflicted with arthritis, or one out of every eleven people. *The Statistical Abstract of the United States* published after the 1970 census counts over 40 million people reporting cases of arthritis. The extent to which these are truly diagnosed cases is not determined. In any case, it is a significant crippling disease.

There are two forms of arthritis: osteoarthritis and rheumatoid arthritis. Osteoarthritis is generally non-inflammatory, a disorder of the movable joints characterized by deterioration and abrasion of the articular cartilege and the formation of new bone at the joint surfaces. Mild to severe disability may appear gradually with advancing years. Rheumatoid arthritis is the most serious form of the disease. It is very painful and crippling. It is systemic in that it affects the whole body. It will affect primarily the joints, but also the lungs, skin, blood vessels, muscles, spleen, heart, and even the eyes. Women are affected by arthritis three times more often than men.

Arthritis occurs throughout the life span, even affecting children; but it must be considered one of the major detrimental changes of old age. It is a major factor in the design of all spaces and artifacts that the aging will use. Movement, strength, and flexibility are curtailed with even mild cases of arthritis. It affects the shoulders, cervical area of the spine, knees, hips, lumbar area, and the interphalangal joints of the fingers. This last area of affliction greatly affects the elderly person's ability to grasp, control, and grip. Manipulating controls, moving objects, negotiating pathways in environments, and other tasks that were performed readily and easily in youth now become painful, difficult, and time consuming. Although movement should be restrained and limited so as not to aggravate the condition, overresting or too much caution may advance the disease. Control and motion are also seriously affected when arthritis affects the

ANTHROPOMETRICS OF TWO AGE GROUPS					
Left Column is 5th. Percentile, Right is 95th. Percentile					
Dimensions in inches	35 - 44 Yrs.		75 - 79 Yrs.		Sex
Erect Standing Hgt.	64.2	71.7	61.3	69.5	Men
	59.6	66.6	55.3	64.5	Women
Weight	134	207	107	191	Men
	109	184	95	178	Women
Erect Sitting Hgt.	33.3	37.7	31.8	36.1	Men
	31.5	35.4	28.1	34.0	Women
Normal Sitting Hgt.	31.9	36.0	29.8	35.2	Men
	30.1	34.3	27.1	32.8	Women
Knee Hgt.	19.8	23.3	19.0	22.2	Men
	18.0	21.0	17.3	20.7	Women
Elbow Hgt.	7.8	11.3	6.5	10.2	Men
	7.5	10.8	6.4	9.8	Women
Thigh Clearance Hgt.	4.6	6.8	4.1	6.1	Men
	4.2	6 7	4.0	6.1	Women
Upper Leg Length	21.3	24.8	21.0	24.4	Men
	20.5	24.0	19.9	23.5	Women
Popliteal Length	17.4	21.1	17.0	20.8	Men
	17.1	20.7	17.0	19.9	Women
Popliteal Height	15.6	18.8	15.2	17.9	Men
	14.0	17.0	13.5	16.9	Women
Elbow to Elbow	14.1	19.2	14.0	18 7	Men
	12.5	18.2	13.1	18.1	Women
Seat Width	12.4	15.6	12.1	14.9	Men
	12.4	16.5	12.2	16.5	Women

Data Extracted From: Weight, Height, & Selected Body Dimensions of Adults - 1960 - 62 (U.S. Public Health Service)

FIGURE 2
Anthropometrics of two age groups. This chart is a comparison of cross-sectional data on two age groups. It portrays distinct differences that must be accounted for in the design process. Generalized "averages" or percentile "ranges" are ineffective data when a specific age group is the user population of a given facility or product.

hip. Motion is seriously curtailed and the gait in walking is restrained.

By the time people reach 90 years of age, about 98 percent of them will have some form and degree of arthritis. This statistic does not impress at first glance, but consider that in the last 10 years the population over 100 years of age increased by 1200 percent. There are over 100,000 people over the age of 100 in the United States today.

Weight changes and changes in height and other dimensions of the body are *anthropometric* characteristics. The statistics representing population differences in anthropometric dimensions are cross-sectional data (see Figure 2). They do not really reflect changes that occur over the life span. What is represented are two different, and in many ways distinct, populations, which are mathematically balanced with all the other populations to become an "average" man and woman. In many respects, the designer has no choice except to use this information in the usual homogenized form. Typically, the designer selects a range of statistical sizes from the fifth percentile to ninety-fifth upon which to base his designs. The problem is that no one person, including the aging person, is truly represented in the final numbers. Unfortunately, the Dreyfuss information presently in use by most industrial designers and others in the fields in design does not include the aging population as a percentage of the population. Public health information does include this information, but the rendering is not in a form conducive to use by designers. The *Human-Scale* publication by Diffrient et al. makes an attempt to integrate some information on handicaps and on the anthropometrics of the elderly.

While the anthropometric data represented are cross sectional, they do reflect some of the physiological changes that occur with age. There are weight gains and then losses over the years; height is reduced and sitting posture is critically affected in many adults. There are qualitative changes as well. The mass of the body shifts. In women, fat deposits shift to the upper thighs. Obesity occurs with some frequency with advancing age, especially among women. The trunk, upper thighs, and breasts may acquire more fatty tissue (Skerlj et al., 1953, p. 450).

MAJOR ORGANS: THE AGING HEART, LUNGS, AND KIDNEYS

Heart

At rest, the aged heart has a slower rate and lower output than that of the young heart. Approximately 70 percent of the output is maintained in the old heart over what it was in the prime of life. It should be remembered, however, that the blood supply remains adequate even though reduced. Body organs in general are "overdesigned" for their purpose, possessing a capacity well above that necessary to sustain health. The importance of reduced output is that under stress there is less reserve to retrieve homeostasis. The heart is also not as able to process as much oxygen within its own tissue. Blood pressure is higher. These affects combined make the heart under stress very susceptible to malfunction.

Here, again, the effects of the environment and culture are important factors in the maintenance of a healthy heart. Excessive smoking and drinking of alcohol, intake of fats in the diet, and lack of exercise are factors influencing the health of the heart. Many Americans are reaching old age with substantially weakened or overloaded hearts because of these factors. Advances in the cure of heart disease are likely to do little to prolong life, but will greatly increase the number of middle-aged people surviving to become old—meaning that a greater number of older people will be living with weak hearts.

Lungs

The lungs' ability to oxygenate the blood decreases with age. At 75, a man's lungs may have half the capacity for oxygenating blood of a man of 20 years. Again, the quantity is sufficient at rest but under stress is inadequate. Another way to view this aspect of lungs capacity is that under stress the aging muscles will require the aging lungs to intake twice as much oxygen to process. Yet, there is less lung capacity, decreased elasticity of the lungs and chest walls, and probably decreases in the number of cells to oxygenate.

Environmental and cultural factors are just as important to the health of the lungs as to the heart. The overeating of fats and proteins, smoking, and drinking are very influential in the health of the lungs.

Kidneys

Like the heart and lungs, the kidneys are also diminished in capability with age. There is a general reduction of cells in the kidneys to half of those available at the age of 30. In the normal process of aging, however, there is a concurrent reduction of cellular structures and tissue in the other portions and

organs of the body, resulting in less waste to be processed. About half the blood is pumped to the kidney in advanced years than was pumped in younger years.

Kidney failure can occur when there is an overload or a disease present in the organism. The overload condition might be either abnormal stress or some external source of stimulus—drugs or a change in diet, as examples.

One of the more distressing discomforts and ailments with advanced years is malfunction or disease in the urinary tract. The elderly who are afflicted with this type of condition are subject to feelings of social distress as well as personal discomfort. If urinary tract infection can be checked in an aging person, very often urinary incontinence can be thwarted. Likewise, drugs must be prescribed judiciously, because the "management" drugs often used in nursing homes frequently result in incontinence. The health care specialist who trades physiological well-being for a more docile recipient of medical treatment is very often trading away long-term benefits for short-term results. The very powerful drugs used in the nursing home have only short-term effectiveness. In the final analysis, the patient is not only the management problem he or she was initially, but the drugs have also reduced organic functioning, which will not be alleviated during the patient's lifetime.

Research in progress conducted by L. Bruce Archer and his colleagues at the Royal College of Art in London on the design of special equipment for the home to maintain the elderly as independents shows that incontinence frightens and confuses the children of aging parents (personal communication, 1975). Although this may be the only malady the aging family member has contracted with age, there is no way for the children to take care of the parent's needs or handle the quantity of wash and general cleaning that results. Archer's team is currently working on special products designed for the home to help with this problem.

Incontinence in general seems to be the chief design criterion for seating and other space and artifact design for nursing homes. Incontinence is a design problem largely because the medical, physiological, and rehabilitation techniques available to alleviate incontinence are not used effectively.

THE AGING SENSORY ORGANS

Designers who have been concerned with problems of the aged have concentrated their efforts on two areas: handicaps and sensory deprivation. Handicaps, which will be discussed following this section, are of interest to designers primarily because of mobility. Sensory deprivation is of interest because of communication. Included in this area are sight, hearing, taste, touch, smell, and temperature sensitivity. Out of this group, sight and hearing have received the major share of attention, because if one cannot see or hear very well then the environment becomes very difficult to interpret and negotiate unless very specialized. It will be shown that, when sensory deprivation is the general block or barrier to regular communications, "redundancy" of communications, using several channels of communication to reinforce content, is a possible and practical solution.

Communications used to help negotiate an environment are as overt as a sign saying exit or as subtle as discrete audible shifts in background noise to clue a person about passage from one place to another. This type of communications is referred to as cuing. Simply defined, a cue is a stimulus that provides information about an environment to its user. Cues are usually associated with direction or place. In a broader context, cues also provide information to the user of an environment about his well-being.

With regard to well-being, the personalization of patient rooms in nursing homes (pictures on walls, personal items on shelves, etc.) is a sign that the patient still maintains some if not total control over the space he or she inhabits. Where there is a recognized but undefined connection between the will to live and health, the surround an elderly person creates for himself or herself is most important. The objects themselves may be odd choices to younger adults. Their value lies in their stimulus and meanings beyond the decorative value of the artifact. A recurring choice of object in this category is the door from the dwelling the elderly resident lived in prior to entrance into the nursing home. The same story is told every time: the door acts as a stimulus (cue) for memories about the friends and acquaintances who entered their homes.

Sight

The visual channel is the most utilized mechanism for receiving and interpreting information. As everyone ages, the lens of the eye is subject to increasing opacity (crystalline lens). The lens also becomes thicker and yellowish (Corso, 1971). This gradual change can impair the perception of colors, especially the perception of blues, greens, and purples (Braun, 1959; Gilbert, 1957). Depth perception can also be subject to acute loss with age (Hoffman et al., 1959). There is also a crazing or wearing of the cornea with age.

As with other organs, the sensory organs are susceptible to diminished capability and disease relating to other bodily changes. Diabetes, hypertension, and artereosclerosis can often affect vision and are frequently responsible for maladies of the eye. The same effects can be traced to diseases of other organs and parts of the body on the other sensory organs.

Macular disease accounts for about 45 percent of the eye problems of the aged. Cataracts account for about 33 percent. Macular disease refers to a pathology of the center vision (macula) of the eye. The ability to discriminate detail, fine print, faces, and the like, is diminished (Figure 3). When the mid or far periphery of the eye is affected, "tunnel vision" occurs. This is a severe handicap in the negotiation of space. Side vision is critical in perceiving motion. Seeing an oncoming person or automobile is difficult. Peripheral vision is a key warning system employed almost unnoticeably by the human organism. The loss of warning devices places the aged person in danger when young adults would be quite safe.

The term cataract is used to classify lens opacity, mentioned previously, that has reached a critical level. All lens opacity is the formation of cataracts. When opacity is such that vision is seriously impaired, the lens can be removed surgically. This treatment is not advisable in the largest majority of cases where opacity is occurring. The trade off of clearer vision and susceptibility to glare from the wearing of heavy-lens glasses should only be done where vision is seriously impaired.

Glaucoma is an increase of intraocular pressure. Ninety percent of all cases occur in people over 40. Advanced cases result in blindness.

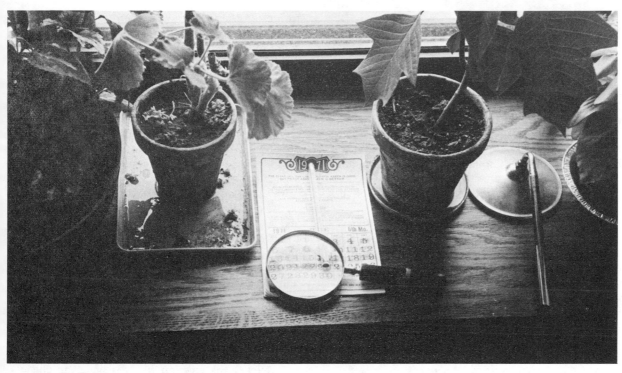

FIGURE 3
Clues to vision problems. (Photo: John Kelsey and Robert Steinbugler.)

While there are vision losses over the age of 50 in the majority of the population, serious loss as described herein affects people beyond the age of 70. This is indeed a critical influence on the design of nursing home space, because the majority of people who reside in nursing homes are over the age of 70.

Hearing

Hearing losses are sustained in a sizable proportion of the population after the age of 40 (Birren, 1964). The critical function of hearing is the continual monitoring of the environment around the listener. Sounds relate the listener to his environment, provide warning signals, and can help isolate the listener from his surroundings. Hearing speech is a secondary aspect of the function of hearing. Interpersonal communications is important and should be promoted in whatever environment the elderly inhabit. However, the discrimination of words, the framing of words, and the distinguishing of voice sounds from background noise become difficult as aging progresses. Many elderly residents of institutional settings want to communicate with others and feel thwarted by environmental as well as social barriers. Still other prefer isolation.

Problems that can inhibit normal hearing can be caused by (1) a conductive hearing loss at the external and middle ear, (2) a sensory loss due to dysfunction of the inner ear or auditory nerve, (3) a combination of these. It is important to note that sheer volume or amplification of total sound will not increase message reception in many cases (Sunturia and Price, 1971).

An important factor involved in poor hearing of speech in referred to as "flat loss." This is the loss of hearing at all frequencies of sound. Speech falls between 500 and 3000 cycles per second. Another form of loss is when hearing is impaired at selected or different frequencies. When there is a loss at high frequencies and none at low, vowel sounds are heard and consonant sounds are not heard. Words such as "hog," "bog," "sog," and "fog" become "og." No amount of amplification will correct this impairment.

Presbycusis, a progressive hearing loss, actually begins early in life with decrements occurring in the high-pitched range of sound. Gradually, the middle range of hearing is affected. This progressive loss forces the listener to rely on visual clues and lip reading to overcome the distortions in sound.

There is now increased attention being paid to hearing losses in recent years for two reasons: (1) the urban–industrial environment has become very noisy and is affecting a greater number of people to a measurable degree, and (2) young people have acquired listening habits that are serious impairments to hearing. It is indeed a disturbing prospect to consider that greater and greater numbers of people will approach and achieve old age in this country with impaired hearing, beyond the normal percentages and beyond the normal levels of impairment.

Tactility, Taste, Smell, and Temperature Sensitivity

All these senses are diminished with age, but the precise measure of their decline has not been made. The precise manner of the decline of effectiveness of these senses is difficult to describe. Research is inconclusive, but a gross representation is clearly that there is a numbing, a loss of precise discrimination. There is less sensitive feel, lessening of the ability to distinguish sweet from salty tastes, where these discriminations are fine, and less realization of slight rises in temperature of the surroundings. These statements must be regarded with caution. Few data exist to show the precise nature of change or quantity of change, much less the qualitative aspects of these changes.

Many questions are still unanswered about organic and physiological changes. Warm to tropical climates provide the chance of stress in high heat and organic-homeostatic imbalance. Yet aging people are attracted to Florida, Arizona, and Southern California in large numbers to avoid the discomfort of cold weather conditions in temperate zones. Is this advisable in the light of present knowledge? Is "clutter" part of the cuing mechanism attached to well-being or is it a need for a more tactile environment? Older people are more apt to move closer to others when conversing. Is this an attempt to recognize through touch and smell as well as sight? What foods appeal to this group of people, and is some weight loss due to an ambivalent attitude toward the taste, texture, and familiarity of available foods?

An introductory statement in this section referred to the communications in an environment being overt and subtle. People often develop a sense of something through sources they cannot identify. The sensory channels are always open and providing information to the human organism. Sensory deprivation not only affects the reactions and interpretations of overt signals through the expected channels of sight and hearing, but also affects the more subtle traces of information constantly utilized by the organism. If the quantity and quality of these signals change, shouldn't the designer, planner, and nursing home staff expect the reaction to these signals to change?

SUMMARY

Human factors information about the nature of aging and the aged is still unfolding. There is much to be done to develop a more comprehensive picture of the process and the people. The information given here is a synthesis. This information has not been clearly developed by research to the fullest extent and a great deal remains to be accomplished. However, designers and those concerned about developing physical plants for institutional purposes must recognize the differences of the aging from other generations. This is not always clearly in evidence when present-day nursing home structures are given even cursory investigation.

Aging is not an arbitrary designation but a physiological fact of life. No one ages at the same rate as another person. It is possible for someone in their 80's to have normal or extraordinary vision, for instance. It is important to recognize that people over the age of 65 are not a homogeneous and monolithic group. They are as varied physiologically as they may be intellectually or socially. Generally, the population over 65 has health problems. Fully 80 percent have some chronic condition. This ranges from diminishing eyesight to advanced rheumatoid arthritis and other disabling conditions. Nursing home populations will have anywhere from 20 to 80 percent of their numbers nonambulatory, either in wheelchairs or geriatric wheelchairs (the geriatric wheelchair cannot be moved by the patient and has cushioned seats). In other words, depending on the level of care in the nursing home, there is either a sizable minority who must be accommodated as wheelchair users or an overwhelming majority.

The nursing home has been created for the physiological support of infirm elderly people. This means that 4 to 5 percent of the elderly over 65 years of age require the type of support generally found in these environments. If the concept held of aging is that it is adjustive and dynamic, these environments must be designed and maintained to support psychological and sociological needs as well. Most nursing home personnel today view this responsibility as secondary, and most physical plants are designed in such a way as to preclude the psychological adjustment needs of this population. This dynamic relationship between the psychological and physiological means that it is actually impossible to separate the two aspects of human development.

Carrying this idea of psychological and sociological accommodation one step further, designers and planners of nursing home facilities must recognize the fact that the populations of these institutions are going to have an overwhelming majority of women as residents. Census statistics and institutional research studies clearly show that the ratio of women to men in these advanced years is approaching ten to one. It is not uncommon to find that, out of 100 patients in a nursing home, only a few will be men. The predominant common denominator for most facilities will be the needs of women.

Discussion of these needs should be more substantive than a cursory summation at the end of physiological design constraints. The important implications are social and psychological as well as physiological. It would be wise for designers and planners to consult diligently with the women who will be residing in the nursing homes and to make sure that women designers are moved into positions of authority in the design process when facilities are going to be built (the largest proportion of designers are men, and a conscious effort would have to be made to move women into the planning and design activities).

REFERENCES

Balchum, Oscar J. "The Aging Respiratory System." In *Working with Older People*, vol. IV, Austin B. Chinn (ed.). U.S. Public Health Service, Department of Health, Education, and Welfare, Rockville, Md., 1971, pub. no. 1459, pp. 113–123.

Birren, James E. *The Psychology of Aging*. Englewood Cliffs, N.J.: Prentice-Hall, Inc., 1964. Chapter 4, "Special Senses and Perception."

Braun, Harry W. "Perceptual Processes." In *Handbook of Aging and the Individual*, James E. Birren (ed.). Chicago: University of Chicago Press, 1959, pp. 543–561.

Chinn, Austin B. "Metabolism, Homeostasis and the Older Patient." In *Working with Older People*, vol. IV, Austin B. Chinn (ed.). U.S. Public Health Service, Department of Health, Education, and Welfare, Rockville, Md., 1971, pub. no. 1459, pp. 241–249.

Comfort, A. *The Biology of Senescence*. London: Routledge & Kegan Paul Ltd., 1956.

Corso, John F. "Sensory Processes and Age Effects in Normal Adults." *Journal of Gerontology*, 26, no. 1 (1971), pp. 90–105.

De Beauvoir, Simone. *The Second Sex*. New York: Alfred A. Knopf, Inc., 1957.

Diffrient, Nils, et al. *HumanScale*. Boston: The M.I.T. Press, 1974.

Dreyfuss, Henry. *The Measure of Man*. New York: Whitney Library of Design, 1966.

Freehafer, Alvin A. "Injuries to the Skeletal System of Older Persons." In *Working with Older People*, vol. IV, Austin B. Chinn (ed.) U.S. Public Health Service, Department of Health, Education, and Welfare, Rockville, Md., 1971, pub. no. 1459, pp. 180–193.

Frohse, Franz, Max Brodel, and Leon Schlossberg. *Atlas of Human Anatomy*. New York: Barnes & Noble, Publishers, 1968.

Gerard, R.W. "Aging and Organization." In *Handbook of Aging and the Individual*, James E. Birren (ed.). Chicago: University of Chicago Press, 1959.

Gilbert, Jeanne G. "Age Changes in Color Matching." *Journal of Gerontology*, 12 (1957), pp. 210-215.

Gordon, Dan M. "Visual Impairments in the Older Patient." *Journal of the American Geriatrics Society*, 15, no. 11 (1967), pp. 1025-1030.

——. "Eye Problems of the Aged." In *Working with Older People*, vol. III, Austin B. Chinn (ed.). U.S. Public Health Service, Department of Health, Education, and Welfare, Rockville, Md., 1971, pub. no. 1459, pp. 28-37.

Grob, David. "Common Disorders of Muscles in the Aged." In *Working with Older People*, vol. III, Austin B. Chinn (ed.). U.S. Public Health Service, Department of Health, Education, and Welfare, Rockville, Md., 1971, pub. no. 1459, pp. 156-162.

——. "Prevalent Joint Diseases in Older Persons." In *Working with Older People*, vol. III, Austin B. Chinn (ed.). U.S. Public Health Service, Department of Health, Education, and Welfare, Rockville, Md., 1971, pub. no. 1459, pp. 163-171.

Harris, Raymond. "Special Features of Heart Disease in the Elderly Patients." In *Working with Older People*, vol. III, Austin B. Chinn (ed.). U.S. Public Health Service, Department of Health, Education, and Welfare, Rockville, Md., 1971, pub. no. 1459, pp. 81-102.

Havighurst, R. J. *Human Development and Education*. New York: David McKay Company, Inc., 1953, pp. 117-136.

Hoffman, C. S., A. Cooper-Price, E. S. Garrett, and W. Rothstein. "Effect of Age and Brain Damage on Depth Perception." *Perceptual and Motor Skills*, 9 (1959), pp. 283-286.

Horvath, S. M., C. E. Radcliffe, B. K. Hutt, and G. B. Spurr. "Metabolic Responses of Old People to a Cold Environment." *Journal of Applied Physiology*, no. 8 (1955), pp. 145-148.

Jaffe, Jack M. "Common Lower Urinary Tract Problems in Older Persons." In *Working with Older People*, vol. IV, Austin B. Chinn (ed.). U.S. Public Health Service, Department of Health, Educa-tion, and Welfare, Rockville, Md., 1971, pub. no. 1459, pp. 141-148.

Kahn, Alvin J., and J. Snapper. "Medical Renal Diseases in the Aged." In *Working with Older People*, vol. IV, Austin B. Chinn (ed.). U.S. Public Health Service, Department of Health, Education, and Welfare, Rockville, Md., 1971, pub. no. 1459, pp. 131-140.

Kleemeier, Robert W. "Behavior and the Organization of the Bodily and External Environment." In *Handbook of Aging and the Individual*. James E. Birren (ed.). Chicago: University of Chicago Press, 1959, pp. 400-437.

Klopper, Walter G. *The Interpersonal Theory of Adjustment. Contributions to the Psychobiology of Aging*. Robert Kastenbaum (ed.). New York: Springer Publishing Company, Inc., 1964, pp. 179-185.

Kuhlen, Raymond G. "Aging and Life Adjustment." In *Handbook of Aging and the Individual*, James E. Birren (ed.). Chicago: University of Chicago Press, 1959, Part VI.

Krag, C. L., and W. B. Kountz. "Stability of Body Function in the Aged." *Journal of Gerontology*, no. 5 (1950), pp. 227-235. I. Effect of exposure of the body of cold; no. 7 (1952), pp. 61-70. II. Effect of exposure of the body to heat.

Kubler-Ross, Elizabeth. *On Death and Dying*. New York: Macmillan Publishing Co., Inc., 1969.

Lawton, M. Powell. "Ecology and Aging." In *Spatial Behavior of Older People*, L. D. Pastalan and D. H. Carson (eds.). Ann Arbor, Mich.: University of Michigan Press, 1970, pp. 40-67.

Locke, Simeon. "Neurological Disorders of the Elderly." In *Working with Older People*, vol. IV, Austin B. Chinn (ed.). U.S. Public Health Service, Department of Health, Education, and Welfare, Rockville, Md., 1971, pub. no. 1459, pp. 45-48.

Lutwak, Leo. "Metabolic Disorders of the Skeleton in Aging." In *Working with Older People*, vol. IV, Austin B. Chinn (ed.). U.S. Public Health Service, Department of Health, Education, and Welfare, Rockville, Md., 1971, pub. no. 1459, pp. 172-179.

Masters, William H., and Virginia E. Johnson. *Human*

Sexual Response. Boston: Little, Brown and Company, 1966, Chapters 15 and 16, pp. 223–270.

Murray, M. Patricia, Kory, Ross C., and Clarkson, Bertha H. "Walking Patterns in Healthy Old Men." *Journal of Gerontology*, 24, no. 1 (1969), pp. 169–178.

Parker, Willard. "Homeostasis." In *Personality in Middle and Late Life*, Bruce Neugarten (ed.). New York: Atherton Press, 1964, pp. 321–324.

——. "Hearing and Age." *Geriatrics*, 24, no. 4 (1969), pp. 151–157.

Pastalan, Leon A. "Privacy Preferences Among Relocated Institutionalized Elderly." *EDRA5*, Environmental Research Association, Inc., 1974.

Public Health Service. *Vital and Health Statistics*. U.S. Department of Health, Education, and Welfare, 1965, pub. no. 1000, series 11, no. 8.

Reichenbach, Maria, and Ruth Anna Mathers. "The Place of Time and Aging in the Natural Sciences and Scientific Philosophy." In *Handbook of Aging and the Individual*, James E. Birren (ed.). Chicago: University of Chicago Press, 1959, pp. 43–80.

Selected Height, Weight and Body Dimensions. U.S. Public Health Service, 1969.

Shock, N. W. "Aging of Homeostatic Mechanisms." In *Cowdrey's Problems of Aging*, Lansings (ed.). Baltimore, Md.: The Williams & Wilkins Company, 1952, pp. 415–446.

Skerlj, B., J. Brozek, and E. E. Hunt. "Subcutaneous Fat and Age Changes in Body Build and Body Form in Women." *American Journal of Physical Anthropology*, no. 11 (1953), pp. 577–600.

The Statistical Abstract of the United States, 1970 Census, 1974 Census. Washington, D.C.: Superintendent of Documents.

Sunturia, Ben H., and Lloyd L. Price. "Otolaryngological Problems in the Geriatric Patient." In *Working with Older People*, vol. IV, Austin B. Chinn (ed.). U.S. Public Health Service, Department of Health, Education, and Welfare, Rockville, Md., 1971, pub. no. 1459, pp. 113–123.

U.S. Census of Population. Washington, D.C.: U.S. Department of Commerce, U.S. Government Printing Office.

CULTURAL, SOCIAL, AND PSYCHOLOGICAL ASPECTS OF NURSING HOME RESIDENCY

The literature is prodigious in the area of social gerontology, and to expand the periphery beyond that of an environmental focus would mean covering so much written material as to distract the reader from the essential thrust of this document. Even so, a glossy and in some ways superficial impression of available material can be created so that the appetite is whetted without destroying the sense of taste for the wealth of information that does exist.

There is, however, a cautionary note to be sounded. A great deal has been written, probably because of the many professionals who have an interest in social gerontology. But much knowledge, indeed the greater share of knowledge about how environments affect people, needs to be established through research and documentation. Far too many of the documents prepared in this field begin or end with the phrase, "little is known," or "a great deal remains to be done." The curious investigator surveying the amount already published wonders just how much work it will take.

In 1971, the American Psychological Association sponsored the assembly of documents on adult development and aging in the field of psychology. The resulting publication (Lawton and Eisdorfer, 1971) is an excellent compendium of the state of the art. The

editors make two key summary statements about special housing for the elderly and the institutional environment:

1. Many of the psychological difficulties of the older person appear to result from a lack of environmental supports, rather than from the aging process per se. Inadequate housing, deterioration of older neighborhoods, antitherapeutic institutions, poorly located services, inadequate transportation, and architectural barriers to mobility may act directly upon the emotional and physical states of any vulnerable individual, old or young.
2. For some older people, the most appropriate place for care is a total custody institution. In contrast to the usual attitude of hopelessness about such patients, research has repeatedly demonstrated the effectiveness of rehabilitative and therapeutic programs in aiding institutionalized aging patients to live more satisfying lives in the institution and frequently enabling them to return to the community (pp. x and xi).

Zubin's (pp. 5-6) brings out two important factors in the development of older people. First, that the learning rate is slower but that this does not indicate a lack of capacity to learn. Second, self-image and self-esteem decline with age; elderly people generally believe they are less than what they were, and this affects their perception of their own capabilities, which may be unwarranted. Neugarten (p. 313) poses the question: "Is the organism biologically programmed only toward maturity, with post maturity changes to be regarded as haphazard? Or is it programmed toward death and decline?" Lawton and Nahemow (pp. 619–666) seek to establish the concept that like all natural organisms, man, especially in advanced years, reacts in a system of interdependencies. He adapts to his environment and makes his environment adapt to him if he has the power to do so. Changes that come in too rapid a succession or come when the organism is in a state of greater than normal dependency can mean a loss of a clearly established value base or persuasability—a dangerous acquiesence found in many institutionalized elderly people.

Cultural aspects are important to note briefly, at least to clarify why many elderly find themselves alone at advanced age and also to point out some myths about aging and the American society. There is an often repeated myth concerning the American family that has a conditioning influence upon the uninitiated dealing with problems of the aging for the first time. The myth is the "extended family." Sometimes called the "three-generation" family, this concoction harkens the unwary sentimentalist to a far better past when grandmother and grandfather lived with their children and their children's children under the same roof in an agrarian setting, growing their own food and working together (Kira, 1958; reprinted, 1968). As the myth has it, the wisdom and knowledge of the elders was passed on through a cooperative venture, through living together and taking care of one another. Nursing homes were unnecessary, so the myth goes, because the respected elders were taken care of in the home.

Superficial investigation of life expectancy of even 40 years ago will show that people usually didn't live long enough to see their grandchildren in great numbers. In 1950, only one out of five elderly persons lived with relatives and only 15 percent of the total population lived in rural settings. Even from the beginning of the settling of the United States, expansion

and mobility drew families apart; America did not wait for the automobile to become mobile. In rural America, families often separated into different dwellings on the same property. These were referred to as "granny cottages."

In Europe, where there was less or no expansion over the same period and land was dear, the grandfather controlled the family through land ownership. The kinship ties in Europe are no stronger than they are in America, and as industry drew young people away from the farms or socialism wrested land from the farmer, the ties were broken—perhaps more properly, given up with little reluctance.

Certainly, three-generation extended families have existed and do exist today. However, they were never a powerful social force and never really existed in great numbers.

Since the greater share of the American population has been born after the turn of the century, the real social and cultural forces impinging upon the family and the elderly members of society have been the urbanized setting and all its manifestations of working roles, life style, and ecological constraints. If the rural setting and its housing at least provided the room for additional members of the family, urban housing has not been so spacious (Kira, 1958). Also, when people have aged and retired in the past and their income has become reduced or fixed, there has sometimes been economic pressure to move from large dwellings in socially secure neighborhoods to smaller units where the elderly are not provided with a sense of personal physical and psychological security (Burgess, 1954).

Perhaps one of the more important aspects of the mythological attitude concerning the elderly is retirement, the force that defines who is an aging person in the first place and is largely the determinant setting the sixty-fifth year as an arbitrary cutoff between middle age and elderliness. There is a general attitude that retirement—the act itself or the force in society—is responsible for loss of purposefulness among the elderly, and also possible losses in physiological health and especially psychological well-being. In part, the difficulty in coping with aging is the general persistence among older adults of the belief that they are not old but "young" (Tibbitts, 1960).

In Streib and Schneider (1971), there is evidence through one of the few longitudinal studies of retiring adults that retirement, in and of itself, is not responsible for a loss of purpose nor is it responsible for physiological or psychological decline. First, retirement as a discernible transition point in an aging person's life can only be readily established in industrial societies. *Industrial societies have lower mortality rates than agrarian societies.* Also, in the past two or three decades, more people are reaching retirement at earlier ages, in healthier condition, with more economic latitude, and with higher levels of education. It is quite obvious that as society projects needs to be met in the future, as well as attempts to solve problems presently involving its resources, attempts to correct old-fashioned concepts about retirement must be made.

As the statistics on population and demography show (Brotman, 1970), there are sizable increases in the population living into the seventieth and eightieth years. Thus, most of the advanced-aged population in the future will be quite knowledgeable about retirement and about personal motivation without employment. It is their changing health status concomitant with personal desires about maintaining independence (not the effects of retirement) that molds future concepts about living arrangements and health facilities.

Yet another myth is somewhat attached to the myth about living arrangements and the structure of the family. It has been assumed that the chief manner in which the elderly are placed in nursing homes is by children who place them there. Children do place their parents in nursing homes, but it in no way represents a majority of the placements. "Extended care facilities," which are facilities meant to provide a level of recuperation below intensive care prices, admit elderly patients after they have been in a hospital. Because most of these facilities are essentially nursing homes, the method of entrance must be considered part of the variety of methods of placement. As stated in the beginning, there are many ways to enter a nursing home, but few ways to leave it.

With the development of a greater variety of managed, custodial care, infirmary, and other types of facilities for the aging, including apartments for the independent elderly, there is a plethora of means,

forces, people, health situations, fears and other devices that direct the aging toward an institutional end point. Often, the segregated, managed, socially oriented facility with the finest intended goals for continued independence is the first step in the conditioning process leading toward institutionalization.

A digression at this point is worthwhile. America is not headed toward less institutionalization, but more. From birth to death, Americans are becoming more reliant on institutions to provide for their needs. Day care for infants is available from six in the morning to six at night. Nursery schools are very popular; secondary schools and elementary schools are not only educational services but conditioning elements in the life of a child. College continues this dependency; more and more planned communities are available for young adults. Retirement is coming at earlier points in the life span. And so on.

There are a great many reasons for this ominous development of institutional dependency through the life span. Women seek greater freedom to act independently and exercise their talents, and well they should. The desire to acquire the life style held before Americans as a dream forces families toward two working spouses. There is fear that without preschool training the child will not be competitive in the elementary classroom. The future may not just hold quicker and more serious separations of adult generations; there may be a hastening of separation of young children from the family—or no family.

There seem to be trends but no real or clear planning. The consequences of these trends will be with this society long after the reasons for their existence have vanished. Indeed, the consequences may actually be the social structure America lives with by the year 2000.

The culture, or more appropriately the prevailing norms, of this society not only shape attitudes toward the structure of society, but shape the man as well. The effects of habits, both healthy and unhealthy, are part of the socialization of an individual. Diet is a response not only to need, but to what seems a part of the social pattern of eating and drinking. Preferences are learned and are part of response conditioned by what is acceptable in the society as a whole.

Even attitudes and methods of exercise are part of a

culture, not just the result of physiological needs or methods of rehabilitation. In the Eastern cultures, for instance, there is more stress given to "passive" methods of exercise: yoga, the Chinese dance exercises, the ritualism of Islam and Hinduism. Western exercise is active conditioning of the muscles, conditioning of the reflexes, and coordination. The ultimate physical specimen in American society is a hard-hitting, explosive linebacker weighing 260 pounds and needing more protein than an entire Indian village to stay in shape. Although this rather facetious example is an extreme, how different is the majority of reconditioning and rehabilitation programming in nursing homes from the athletic conditioning of a linebacker for the Green Bay Packers?

An elderly man in a chronic care or acute care setting with a broken arm may be put through a physical conditioning program that will overstress his capacity to respond by lifting weights, eating proteins, flexing muscles and joints, and so on. It may be far more appropriate to position the body as in Yoga and reduce protein intake. The previous chapter on the physiological aspects of aging provides ample inferences about why this might be so. These suggestions are not prescriptive, but should be considered. Many rehabilitation programs should be carefully considered before specific application to any given elderly patient. The complications resulting from stressful physiotherapy may be worse than the initial trauma.

Cultural norms or the socialization process contribute to the attitudes of younger generations, to older generations, and to the institutions they have mutually designed. It is safe to say that all generations approach the thought of nursing home life with foreboding, in some cases sufficient foreboding to cause death either upon entry or just before. Yet the value of independence beyond a certain point is questionable.

Pressey and Pressey (1972) give a firsthand accounting of life in a nursing home for two elderly and extremely active people, husband and wife, who have carefully recorded their experiences and kept track of others who either remained independent or chose entry into a residential facility for the aged. Out of 110 contacts, the Pressey's counted two thirds who died over a 15-year period. Their's is a remarkable piece

of work because it is conducted by two researchers who have reached old age—they were both in their 80's—when the work was published. The point of the article is the need for counseling older adults about appropriate settings for their retirement and later years. However, there is also a great deal of insight about the physical environment per se and the influence of the setting on older people. With respect to appropriate choices in later years, the Pressey's state:

The folly of continuing too long in the old home was repeatedly evidenced, as by the widow found there dead by a neighbor, the retired teacher also found dead when a friend's phone calls were unanswered, the widow who became senile and was moved from the homestead by a guardian . . . . Many more . . . not needing institutional care in the narrow stigmatized sense, but also facilities, services, and companionships . . . . Choice(s) made in advance of a crisis (p.363).

The Pressey's go on to describe what they call the "gerontological residency." In another article, Pressey suggests that a nursing home should be a "hospice with counseling" (Pressey, 1973). More of the Pressey's observations will be presented later in the text. Their insights, such as the "corridor neighborhood" found in these facilities, are valuable contributions.

The influence of environment upon the behavior of people as a general area of interest has received a great deal of attention in the past few years. Residential and institutional settings for the aging have commanded a great share of this attention because of the dependency of the elderly upon their surroundings for support. The concept of "corridor neighborhood" is part of a very serious endeavor by designers and behavioral scientists to determine the influence of the physical environment upon the elderly.

In Pressey's (1972) article, the physical nature of the environment is clearly an important part of the concept of corridor neighborhood:

In our wing . . . are three bedroom-and-bath apartments and 15 having also living room and kitchenette, on either side of a corridor one end of which opens on a parking area and the other on a passageway leading to the other similar wings and to the common dining room and room for meetings, games, and movies . . . . Yet, as attractive as our lounge is, most of the time during our first year there it was vacant, and contacts in the corridor and service rooms were little more than a smile and nod in passing . . . . Suddenly, after about a year, a cardiac crisis cut off most of those [other] contacts for

Alice; increasingly our little corridor neighborhood was her world (p. 365).

The Pressey's capsulized a very important aspect of the nature of most environments designed, so to speak, to meet the needs of the aging resident: many attractive lounges or spaces meant for socialization do not function very well for that purpose. Behavioral scientists have observed that the elderly residents of housing projects gather to socialize in areas which were not initially designed to function as socialization areas. Lobbies, the nexus of two corridors, laundry rooms, pharmacy waiting areas, and the like, seem to draw people by virtue of some externalized stimulus (watching others) or where there is a commonality of purpose (getting drugs).

Where there is even greater dependency, such as in the nursing home or infirmary settings, mobility status can determine whether people will use particular spaces. Here, again, externalized stimuli will draw the older patient–resident to areas where there is something to observe or talk about. Nursing stations are veritable watering holes of stimulation in many institutions.

Much more detail will be given on these and other spatial uses and arrangements of spaces in the chapter on planning. The essential point is that these phenomena of behavior have been happening with regularity in hundreds of institutions and residential settings, spurring on the intensity of interest in further study.

Again, the literature on behavior and physical environment relationships is prodigious. Edward T. Hall, an anthropologist, was one of the first to identify "spatial behavior" and give it an identity—proxemics (*The Hidden Dimension*, 1969). Robert Sommer's books, *Personal Space* and *Design Awareness*, explore the evidence of the human organism's attachment to his physical surroundings and also the relationships between the professions that are responsible for the design of man's surroundings. Still others (Canter and Wools, 1969; Combs, 1952; Snygg and Combs, 1959; Craik, 1970; Stea, 1969, Ostrander, 1970; Sanoff, 1969; Barker and Barker, 1961; Ittelson et al., 1970; Patterson, 1974) have provided insights into appropriate methodology for investigating man–environment relationships and have shown the importance of heeding behavioral information prior to designing hardware.

David Canter, in a literature review published in 1972, stated that there are possibly over 1000 documents that relate to research in this area.

Perhaps the single most essential or central work in this area is Pastalan and Carson's *Spatial Behavior of Older People*. The book is a compendium of writings by researchers in this field from a 1968 symposium. Robert Sommer (pp. 25-39) discusses the interaction (or lack of it) of elderly with the institutional spaces they inhabit:

Although new furniture, air conditioners, and a TV had been purchased for the ward, there is no record about what the ladies (patients) said about the change since no one had solicited their opinions before or after . . . . Floor tiles . . . were all the same pattern and ran the same way, making the large lounge . . . look even more institutional . . . . Around several columns there were four chairs, each facing a different direction! The tragedy was not that these arrangements existed but that they were accepted as normal and reasonable throughout the institution.

Pastalan (pp. 88-101) discusses privacy as a necessity, something quite lacking in a great many institutions for the aging. He goes on to delineate four states of privacy established in earlier research by Westin (1967): solitude, intimacy, anonymity, and reserve. There is a discussion of how the overall environment impinges upon the right to privacy and how the aging, in social and physical loss continuum, use environmental props to maintain privacy. Pastalan also states that the "flood of ever increasing numbers of . . . environments for the elderly afford a unique research situation . . . [to] yield valuable comparative data in terms of the various parameters of privacy."

The designer will be both encouraged and dismayed as he wades through the literature in this expanding field. The promise has been great but the delivery of information, in the sense of what Pastalan observed as an opportunity, has not come to pass. There is information to be sure on environment and behavior, but it is not readily transferrable to new design, with the possible exception of arrangements of interiors. In this same compendium, Raymond Studer (pp. 104, 105) contemplates the role of the behavioral scientist in relation to design effort:

He [the behavioral scientist] characteristically deals not with synthesis but *analysis*. The general result, as we know, is a fragmented, disparate, and often conflicting collection of findings and resources.

Robert Sommer (1972) suggests a relationship between disciplines to help overcome the difficulties seen by both designers and behavioral scientists:

The history of professions offers us the lesson that one profession cannot rely on another to evaluate its work . . . . Left to himself, the psychologist is likely to be irrelevant and ineffective in the design fields (p. 94).

Related to the idea of interdisciplinary relationship that Sommer suggests, several behavioral scientists and designers and architects are working on projects with individual design jobs as their results. This eliminates the portentious aspect of most research, that of creating highly glossed theories or information too specific about too few variables to be of value. Organizations have also been created where information can be shared on common ground. The Environmental Design and Research Association (EDRA) is one. The Association for the Study of Man–Environment Systems is another group sharing information.

In summary, the promise of a body of knowledge usable by designers and clearly delineating the social and psychological aspects of environment—especially environments for the aging—is in a seminal stage. The possibility of interdisciplinary design teams is perhaps inevitable, but their formulation and responsibilities remain an "empirical" question, as Sommer has suggested.

There are cultural, social, and psychological determinants involved in the design process to be sure. The designer is often unaware of just how many decisions he makes that are culturally derived; their appropriate interpretation is another matter.

The designer should be encouraged to expand his knowledge about the inputs that behavioral scientists are trying in good faith to make to the design process. The more informed the design community becomes about these attempts, the more cooperation will be attained.

However, as these inputs have been forthcoming, their effect is not only to provide useful information about how environments influence man and the elderly in particular, but also to show that the design process is not the prerogative of a special group of people.

Elderly residents of independent living units to nursing home settings, administrators, nursing staffs, and citizen groups are all part of the design process, either by making demands, providing useful information, or acting as knowledgeable critics. If there is one outstanding benefit from the melange of efforts in this area, it is that the design process has been opened up. That is precisely the effect desired for institutions. If the design process can be "opened" to include the input of people who use the physical environment and products within it, there will be an improvement in the quality of environment and in the process of design as well.

REFERENCES

Barker, R. G. *Ecological Psychology: Concepts and Methods for Studying the Environment of Human Behavior*. Stanford, Calif.: Stanford University Press, 1968.
——, and Louise S. Barker. "The Psychological Ecology of Old People in Midwest Kansas, and Yoredale, Yorkshire." *Journal of Gerontology*, 16 (1961), pp. 144-149.
Brotman, Herman B. *The Older Population: Some Facts We Should Know*. Washington, D.C.: Administration on Aging, 1970.
Burgess, E. W. "Communal Arrangements for Older Citizens." In *Housing the Aged*, Wilma Donahue (ed.). Ann Arbor, Mich.: University of Michigan Press, 1954.
Canter, D. *People and Buildings: A Brief Overview of Research*. Monticello, Ill.: Council of Planning Librarians, Aug., 1972.
——, and R. Wools. *A Technique for the Subjective Appraisal of Building*. (Paper presented at CIE Study Group at Stockholm, June 1969.)
Combs, A. "Intelligence from a Perceptual Point of View." *Journal of Abnormal and Social Psychology*, 47 (1952), pp. 662-673.
Craik, K. H. "Environmental Psychology." In *New Directions in Psychology IV*. New York: Holt, Rinehart and Winston, Inc., 1970.
Hall, Edward T. *The Hidden Dimension*. Garden City, N.Y.: Doubleday & Company, Inc., 1969.

Ittelson, William H., L. G. Rivlin, and H. Proshansky. *Environmental Psychology*. New York: Holt, Rinehart and Winston, Inc., 1970.

Kira, Alexander. *Housing Requirements of the Aged: A Study of Design Criteria*. Ithaca, N.Y.: Housing Research Center, Cornell University, 1958. Reprinted 1968.

Lawton, M. Powell, and C. Eisdorfer (eds.). *The Psychology of Adult Development and Aging*. Washington, D.C.: American Psychological Association, 1971.

——, and Lucille Nahemow. "Ecology and the Aging Process." In *The Psychology of Adult Development and Aging*, M. Lawton and C. Eisdorfer (eds.). Washington, D.C.: American Psychological Association, 1971, pp. 619-666.

Neugarten, Bernice, "Personality Change in Late Life: A Developmental Perspective." In *The Psychology of Adult Development and Aging*, M. Lawton and C. Eisdorfer (eds.). Washington, D.C.: American Psychological Association, 1971, p. 313.

Ostrander, E. *Exploratory Studies of User Reactions to their Near Environment: Free Association Techniques*. Unpublished manuscript. Ithaca, N.Y.: Cornell University, Nov. 10, 1970.

Pastalan, Leon A. "Privacy as an Expression of Human Territoriality." In *Spatial Behavior of Older People*, L. A. Pastalan and D. H. Carson (eds.). Ann Arbor, Mich.: University of Michigan Press, 1970, pp. 89-101.

——, and D. H. Carson (eds.). *Spatial Behavior of Older People*, L. A. Pastalan and D. H. Carson (eds.). Ann Arbor, Mich.: University of Michigan Press, 1970.

Patterson, Arthur H. "Unobtrusive Measures: Their Nature and Utility for Architects." In *Designing for Human Behavior*, J. Lang, C. Burnette, W. Moleski, and D. Vachon (eds.). Stroudsburg, Pa.: Dowden Hutchinson & Ross, Inc., 1974, pp. 261-273.

Pressey, Sidney L. "Age Counseling: Crises, Services, Potential." *Journal of Counseling Psychology*, 1973, pp. 356-360.

——, and Alice Pressey. "Major Neglected Need Opportunity: Old Age Counseling." *Journal of Counseling Psychology*, 20 (1972), pp. 362-366.

Sanoff, H. "Visual Attributes of the Physical Environment." In *Response to Environment*, G. Coates and K. Moffert (eds.). Raleigh, N.C.: Student Publications of the School of Design, North Carolina State University, no. 18, 1969, pp. 37-62.

Snygg, D., and A. Combs. *Individual Behavior: A New Frame of Reference for Psychology*. New York: Harper & Row, Inc., 1959.

Sommer, Robert. *Personal Space*. Englewood Cliffs, N.J.: Prentice Hall, Inc., 1969.

——. *Design Awareness*. New York: Holt, Rinehart and Winston, Inc., 1972.

——. "Small Group Ecology in Institutions for the Elderly." In *Spatial Behavior of Older People*, L. A. Pastalan and D. H. Carson (eds.). Ann Arbor, Mich.: University of Michigan, 1970, pp. 25-39.

Stea, D. "Environmental Perception and Cognition: Toward a Model for Mental Maps." In *Response to Environment*, G. Coates and K. Moffert (eds.). Raleigh, N.C.: Student Publications of the School of Design, North Carolina State University, no. 18, 1969, pp. 62-75.

Streib, Gordon F., and Clement J. Schneider. *Retirement in American Society*. Ithaca, N.Y.: Cornell University Press, 1971.

Studer, Raymond. "The Organization of Spatial Stimuli." In *Spatial Behavior of Older People*, L. A. Pastalan and D. H. Carson (eds.). Ann Arbor, Mich.: University of Michigan, 1970, pp. 102-123.

Tibbitts, Clark. "Origin, Scope and Fields of Social Gerontology." In *Handbook of Social Gerontology*, C. Tibbitts (ed.). Chicago: University of Chicago Press, 1960, pp. 3-26.

Westin, Alan. *Privacy and Freedom*. New York: Atheneum Publishers, 1967.

Zubin, Joseph. "Foundations of Gerontology: History, Training, and Methodology." In *The Psychology of Adult Development and Aging*, M. Lawton and C. Eisdorfer (eds.). Washington, D.C.: American Psychological Association, 1971, pp. 5, 6.

PART III
PLANNING

ASPECTS OF PLANNING THE NURSING HOME FACILITY

The first challenge of accomplishing anything in design is defining the problem. "Nursing home" is a vague term which does not become easier to define even after a great deal of experience is acquired in association with the physical environments and the people who operate them. Ostensibly, a nursing home is a health care facility offering 24-hour skilled nursing observation and care to the "chronically" ill. Chronically ill usually implies aging resident–patients, although this is not necessarily a prerequisite for their existence. The physical plants are not required to have an operating theater or provide other "acute" care services. Most are not required to have a full-time physician. Generally, all are required to have a full-time state licensed administrator, and many apply for and receive federal licensure for construction and subsidy for services such as Medicare.

Beyond this level of definition, it becomes difficult to specify all that is entailed in the makeup of a nursing home. There are variations in the wording of types of nursing homes from state to state and the services vary from place to place. The problem is doubly compounded by the rapid evolution of the "industry."

Only two decades ago, the nursing home was a small facility in general. Today the trend is toward a complex of housing and health care components in a linked continuum from independent living to chronic care infirmaries. Whereas a typical nursing home in the not too distant past held a population of resident–patients below 50, the average today holds nearly 100. Campus-type facilities in urban and suburban settings now have a population nearing 1000 or more aging people. These are often referred to as "retirement communities" or "geriatric centers." Services range from minimal medical and social and rehabilitative offerings to the full gamut of these services, depending on need. The majority (90 percent) of these facilities are profit-making businesses, hence the reference to industry. The smallest percentage are public facilities; the private, nonprofit home is a few percentage points greater than the public facilities.

Indeed, it is difficult to comprehend where independent living and nursing care are separated in a large number of present-day facilities. Frequently, aging people are induced to enter the independent units because of the security provided by having medical facilities adjunct to their residence. The transition from one level of care to another may be so indistinguishable that only the paperwork gives an indication of change. There are instances where geriatric centers have decertified one floor of their facilities to allow transfer of patients in and out to maintain Medicare coverage of their health care expenditures when recovery has not taken the prescribed 90-day period.

Smoothing out transfer may be desirable; the trauma of moves and the concomitant anxiety have been shown to be physiologically harmful to the aging. However, the benefits of aggregating large numbers of aging people in supercomplex efficiency-oriented operations is arguable, and many have been vocal about this trend:

One of the most predominant efforts on the part of those who control the power in nursing homes is in the direction of conceiving of the elderly individual as a "sick person." When the individual is conceived of as a sick organism the facility is structured around a medical model. The individual is referred to as a "patient"; the living areas are labeled "ward"; the workers wear white coats or uniforms, professional labels and jargon take on great significance, the "patient's chart" becomes an administrative financial tool rather than a communication medium for the benefit of the client. There develops an intense preoccupation with filling all the beds; the clients are worked over, medicated and treated in response to physicians' orders. Medical and administrative personnel, whether qualified or not, make decisions about nonmedical and nonadministrative matters.

They literally take over the human and personal affairs of the elderly within the field of their control. Such human matters as privacy, contact with the community, decision making, personal hygiene and appearance, self-directed mobility, the right to be outside, possession of personal belongings, knowledge of one's own financial status, pleasing environmental surroundings, right to information about the plans of professionals become the perogative of many people other than the elderly individual himself (or herself) (Baker, 1973).

Baker has capsulized the feelings of many quite well in this statement. The idea has been explored as well by Baynes (1971). Once the person involved essentially as a client is conceived of as a patient, all manner of freedom can be taken away in the name of health care. The effect is precisely the opposite of rehabilitation.

The core of the geriatric facility is most definitely the nursing home section. The retirement community is less directed toward this area. However, the pervasiveness of the health care atmosphere is unavoidable. To maximize independence, then, requires a reversal. To ensure bona fide rehabilitation, it is es-

sential to minimize the affective state of the health care aura and refrain from taking away control over existence from the aging who are the clients.

Little is to be gained by arguing the viability of the super nursing home or the profit-making incentive in health care. These questions interfere with the thrust of this text. The critical issues at this general level of planning are (1) the various levels of care and independence, and (2) the meaning of "health care facility." The order of residency–health care facilities in a scale of ascending health care service provision is as follows:

1. *Managed public housing.* Public housing is not considered a housing type providing services to the elderly. However, the time is near when the needs of those elderly living in public housing must be met either by internal services or through outreach programs of agencies or health facilities in the same catchment area.
2. *Apartments for the elderly.* Independent living units created and financed by a variety of federal funds and programs. These units would not necessarily have public spaces such as lounges or conglomerate dining facilities, although in later building projects these amenities have been provided.
3. *"Domiciliary" housing units.* This designation refers to independent living units where social services, programs, and conglomerate dining facilities are provided.
4. *Health-related facility (HRF).* A step below that of the 24-hour nursing service found in the next level of care. The concept behind the HRF is that it would serve those elderly who have been rehabilitated in nursing homes. Ideally, it should be open to those who find a need for health care services, but do not need 24-hour care. These people would enter from a private dwelling unit or from apartments or domiciliary units. This area of facility development is quite new.
5. *24-hour skilled nursing home.* A health care facility providing round the clock nursing observation and care, meals, social services, physiotherapy, and other programs. This is the true nursing home.
6. *Extended care facility (ECF).* A designation created through Medicare legislation and funding. A

recuperative setting having the amenities of the 24-hour skilled nursing home, but the potential for more intensive rehabilitation—theoretically. Entrance is allowed after treatment in an acute care hospital when recuperation may be extended, but intensive care space is unwarranted. Extended care facilities were created as an idealistic alternative to the nursing home. Ninety days of recuperation were allowed under the law; then the patient becomes a paying customer. The idealism which promoted this conception was that if the elderly could be rehabilitated they would not need long-term care in a nursing home. Statistical evidence shows that very few of the elderly population entering ECF's are actually rehabilitated and sent home. Many are then forced to pay very high fees to remain or become wards of the state in the ECF's administrative, monetary, health service system.

7. *Geriatric hospital.*   An "acute" care setting where the elderly who have been struck down with an affliction or have suffered an accident can be treated by specialists in geriatric medicine in surroundings conducive to their special needs and recovery rate. Although 50 percent of the patients in U.S. hospitals are over 65, there are practically no geriatric hospitals in the United States.

Two other designations are worth exploring because there is rapid development in conglomerate services offered in a variety of packages.

8. *Retirement community.*   A long-term affiliative organization providing housing and social services in an age-segregated community. The emphasis is on leisure activities and a protected environment. They are often expensive and utilize a variety of financial devices to encourage participation.

9. *Geriatric center.*   A long-term contractual organization providing housing and health care services, as well as social programs. The emphasis is health care. The central triumvirate facilities are usually a 24-hour skilled nursing home, health-related facility, and domiciliary housing.

There are other concepts of facilities for the aging that could be employed, even with existing nursing homes or other types of structures. The British have a system of day care–night care facilities for the aging.

If a person has nowhere to go during the day or lives with someone who works and needs care, these facilities will provide care during the day. The reverse situation for the aging person means the provision of night care. There are outreach programs that could be generated from centers into the community, clinics for health checkups by trained paraprofessionals, roving mobile service centers to locate elderly in need of a variety of services, sharing systems in which the elderly could enter the homes of younger people on a mutual voluntary basis, specialized modules attachable to private housing to permit the elderly to remain at home either intermittently or to prolong their stay, and specialized mobile homes (fully 20 percent of the market for mobile homes is people over the age of 65) (Morris and Woods, 1971) with widened isles and appropriately designed amenities. Any number of alternatives are possible and should be explored to meet the variety of needs that exist.

Turning to issues surrounding the physical environment, the first requirement is that the facility to be studied be viewed as an open system to ensure an open design. Environments can be seen as organisms that parallel the life functions and biological attributes of other living systems. If the physical plant is viewed as a separate entity containing mechanical systems to serve the real functions of the organism, the conception of the facility loses its association with the organism. The word "facility" means the absence of difficulty. To call the building of a health care operation a facility indicates that the structure is allowing something—the functions—to be accomplished with ease.

The functions to be carried out are obviously the wide variety of medical, social, administrative and other facets of the operation. These can be expressed in a simple input-output model describing a sequence, as in Figure 4.

A facility is then people and a physical setting acting in response. There is a direction involved. The wholeness of this model is an environment in the truest ecological sense. The physical setting is not *the* environment, but one environment interacting with others, a subsystem of a larger system. These interacting subsystem environments impart attributes to the facility. This model is expressed in Figure 5.

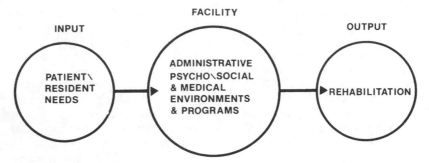

FIGURE 4
Input–output model. When needs and goals are defined, the facility is an agent effecting change, hopefully for the better.

The total facility is a combination of environments that interrelate to make up "facility" in the truest sense. The product of the interaction of these subsystems is goals, attitudes, and attributes. To get to this final stage, however, the interrelated environments produce a three-part set of "atmospheres" or feelings within themselves and throughout the facility, which are either "facilitative" or counterproductive in the scheme of things. The best intentions of an administrative body can be meaningless if proper attention is not given to other components of the system. A facility can seem overly institutional by virtue of a dominant health care atmosphere—one that is conceived of on the supremacy-of-the-giver model. An "institutional" building can be offset by a subdued health care atmosphere and an emphasized rehabilitation service atmosphere. In essence, an appropriate balance of environments and atmospheres must be maintained if the goals defined are to be achieved.

Each component of this system or model is dependent upon the other. The building and artifacts within it are part of the service and the atmosphere. The physical environment can be viewed in a dependency state relying upon the other components as "inputs" vital to its conception and existence. This relationship is expressed in Figure 6.

The key to designing toward openness in a health care facility for the aged is to focus upon the needs, general requirements, and desires of this population from the beginning of the design process. One important facet is to express appropriate concern for the residential qualities of the physical environment, as well as the health care and service aspects of the setting. It would be better to overstress residency vis-à-vis health care in the general qualitative atmosphere in order to prevent institutionalization from becoming predominant esthetically and attitudinally.

A concern for environments with respect to atmospheres, attitudes, and attributes generally leads to studies of behavior. Activities occur within space, and spaces generally derive their designations from the activities that occur within them. Unfortunately, the designations provided as labels in health care facilities are often misapplied or too restrictive. Spivak (1973) developed a set of archetypical behaviors common to all generations and related to "places" within physical settings. With the exclusion of "child bearing" and "nursery," there are 16 archetypical behaviors that are useful in determining the range of possible activities to be allocated space. These are given in Table 1.

If a truly representative facility is to be designed, all the archetypical behaviors mentioned must be accommodated by allocations of space and artifacts to support their existence.

One of the first inclinations in the design process is to allocate a space for each of the archetypical behaviors. A variation of this is to designate a space for prescribed activities and to define the activity according to the space. This is how most codes specify

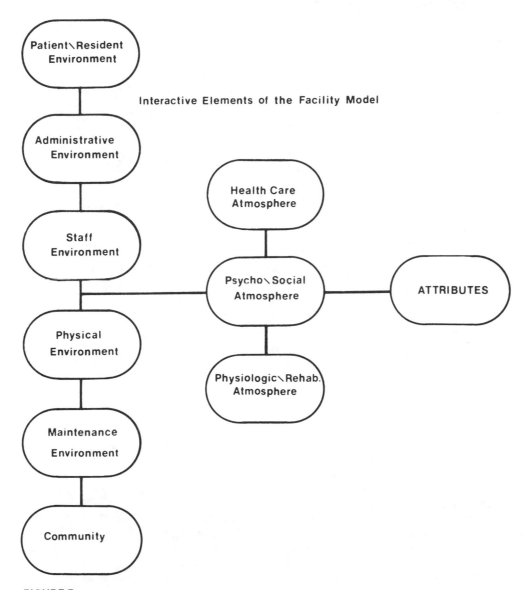

Interactive Elements of the Facility Model

Patient\Resident Environment

Administrative Environment

Staff Environment

Physical Environment

Maintenance Environment

Community

Health Care Atmosphere

Psycho\Social Atmosphere

Physiologic\Rehab. Atmosphere

ATTRIBUTES

FIGURE 5

Interactive elements of the facility model. A "facility" is a collection of environments interacting to produce atmospheres and attributes. The "space" and "objects in space" make up the physical environment, which is *not* the dominating element, by any means. A sound administrative environment and empathetic nursing can make up for substantial physical environmental deficits.

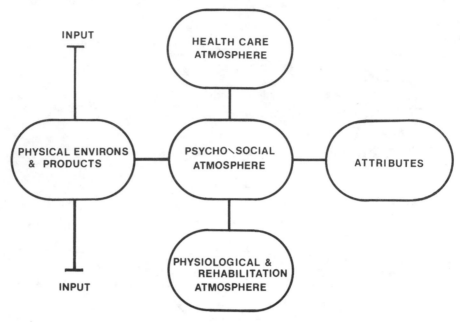

FIGURE 6

Physical environment section. An understanding of the relationship of the physical environment to other components of the facility can be gained by studying use. Other environments
must be seen as contributing to use and therefore become inputs to this research process.

the requirements for a given facility. The object is to accommodate; the effect is to designate regardless of real function or the real requirements.

According to most specifications, the designers, or anyone concerned with the planning and building of health care facilities, spaces are *unifunctional*. That is, spaces are provided for a single designated use: lounges are for relaxing and socializing, dining areas are for eating, and so on. The facts are that spaces are *multifunctional*, serving many requirements—both designated and undesignated, and they will be altered with time and by changes in population. A truly accurate prediction of the use of any given space over the life of a building is impossible and not very useful. It is more important to first realize how many spaces and artifacts are being used now, and to try to facilitate the behaviors that are normal and required for continuation of involvements and existence itself.

The patient-residents of nursing homes normally

have access to 12 distinct spaces within a facility. They do not have either unlimited or unrestricted access to all these areas, but most will use these spaces at least occasionally. Some patient–residents will not use some of these areas at all. These "archetypical" spaces are as follows:

1. Patient-resident room
2. Lounge
3. Corridors
4. Dining rooms
5. Entrance areas and lobbies
6. Activity areas
7. Bathrooms
8. Occupational therapy areas
9. Physiotherapy areas
10. Beauty parlors and barbershops
11. Chapels and worship areas
12. Outside areas and the community

TABLE 1 Common Archetypical Behaviors

Archetype	Descriptive Behavior
Nesting	Elemental protection; protection for nesting activities; retreat from stimulation, aggression, threat, social contact; emotional recuperation.
Sleeping	Sleeping; dreaming.
Mating	Courting rituals; pair bonding; copulation; affectional behavior; communication.
Rehabilitation-healing	Recuperation; care of illness, injury; special rest out of phase with diurnal cycle; reduced stimulation in controlled environment; special ritual; props; instruments; foods; death.
Grooming	Washing; social or mutual grooming.
Nourishment	Eating; feeding; slaking thirst; communication; social gathering.
Excretion	Excreting; territorial marking.
Storing	Hiding of food and other property; storage; hoarding.
Passive activity	Spying; contemplating; meditation; planning; waiting; territorial sentry; watching.
Engaged activity	Motor satisfactions: role testing; role changing; role breaking; fantasy; exercising; creation; discovery; dominance; confirmation; analysis and synthesis.
Locomotion	Perimeter checking; territorial confirmation; motor satisfaction; place changing.
Meeting	Social gathering; communication; dominance confirmation; governing; educating.
Working	Hunting; gathering; earning; building; making.
Competing	Formal agnostic ritual; dominance assertion; ecological competition; interspecies defense; intraspecies defense and aggression; mating competition; conflict.
Learning	Formal education; conditioning; socialization.
Worshiping	Meditation; cosmic awe; mysticism; reverence to deity; moral concern.

Observation studies have been useful in showing the multifunctional aspect of space utilization, and helpful in referencing uses of space according to spatial allocation and designation. If the archetypical behaviors modified from the Spivak writings are cross-referenced in a matrix with specific spaces according to observations made in the research of Koncelik et al. (1972), behaviors occurred in the predominance shown in Figure 7.

The interactions within the matrix of figure 7 should be seen as the more critical behavior related to archetypical spaces within facilities. All 16 behaviors could potentially happen within all spaces. Circled interactions should be viewed as the most important interactions.

Although each of the 12 areas of access make up the substance of the section on spaces to follow, it is worth extracting some generalities about these archetypical spaces at this point. The importance of the patient-resident room cannot be sufficiently stressed. At present the bulk of rooms are designed around the nursing staff, yet the assessments made through observations by many researchers and others show clearly that the *residential* quality is of great importance if not primary importance. Hence, the designation of the occupant as a *patient-resident:* a patient because the occupant receives health care and rehabilitative services; a resident because the occupant *lives* there and should control this space to the maximum degree possible. For every occupant this degree of control is different. Patient-resident connotes a spectrum of independence to a lesser or greater degree.

The patient-resident room is a sanctuary—or should be. *The largest number of patient-resident rooms in any given facility should be private rooms.* The two-bed room presents so many problems as to be detrimental to effective patient-residential control, privacy, and residential quality. The most important attribute of this space should be its "residential" quality and adequate space for socialization on a spontaneous basis. Most present-day nursing home rooms are hospital-like in their character and space allocation. Yet the words most often heard upon entry in a nursing home are that the planners tried to achieve a "home-like" quality or atmosphere. Indeed, this attempt is often sensed in lounges, entry areas, and dining spaces.

▲ Denotes Interaction
◭ Denotes Significant Interaction

	Nesting	Sleeping	Mating	Rehabilitation	Grooming	Nourishment	Excretion	Storing	Passive Activity	Engaged Activity	Locomotion	Meeting	Working	Competing	Learning	Meditation
1. Patient\Resident Rooms	◭	◭	▲	◭	◭	◭	◭	◭	◭	◭	▲	◭	▲	▲	▲	◭
2. Lounges		▲		▲		▲	▲		◭	▲	◭	◭	▲	▲	▲	▲
3. Corridors		▲		◭		▲	▲		◭	◭	◭	◭			▲	▲
4. Dining Rooms				▲		◭			▲	▲	◭			▲	▲	▲
5. Entrance Areas & Lobbies		▲							◭		▲	◭			▲	▲
6. Activities Areas									▲	▲	▲	▲	◭		▲	▲
7. Bathrooms				▲	◭		◭	▲	▲							
8. Occupational Therapy Areas				◭						◭	▲	▲	◭		▲	
9. Physiotherapy Areas				◭						◭	▲	▲	▲	▲		
10. Beauty Parlors\Barber Shops					▲				◭	▲		◭				
11. Chapels & Worship Areas																◭
12. Outside Areas		▲			▲		▲	▲	◭	▲	◭	◭	▲	▲	▲	

FIGURE 7

Place–behavior interaction matrix. Spivak's (1973) behavioral archetypes can be checked in relation to the spaces that are accessible to patient–residents. In this way the functional characteristics of a space can be more realistically assessed. Interactions shown here have been derived from over five years of experience with observation techniques and clearly show the "multifunctionality" of accessible nursing home spaces.

However, when the observant visitor is able to penetrate as far into the facility as the patient rooms, he becomes aware that the "homelike" quality has vanished somewhere along the way. The corridor neighborhood the Pressey's described is in evidence to some degree, but it is hardly the norm of social behavior—nor is it promoted either by staff or by the physical environment.

Figure 8 illustrates that the first five areas of the facility are the essential components of the corridor neighborhood. It is in these areas that the patient–residents will meet their cohorts, deal with staff and administrators, attempt to maintain their self-reliance and dignity, engage in the 16 archetypical behaviors—live and die.

Other areas of the facility are adjunctory and of less importance in the real rehabilitation atmosphere of the physical environment. It is not feasible nor appropriate to suggest that these other spaces, excluding the outside environment, could be eliminated from the overall plan. But it is not unthinkable that these other spaces could be overstressed. Elaborate activity areas, physiotherapy and occupational therapy areas, and the rest could be integrated into the other spaces in a very unobtrusive way. An effort should be made to make the total rehabilitation process part of daily activity and as natural as dining or socializing. Indeed, the predominant thinking on lounge space is to translate square footage into one or two large lounge spaces for the whole facility. This usually means that accessibility for many of the more incapacitated elderly is limited if not fully cut off. Why can't the square footage requirements devoted to lounge space on a per capita or bed number basis be translated into

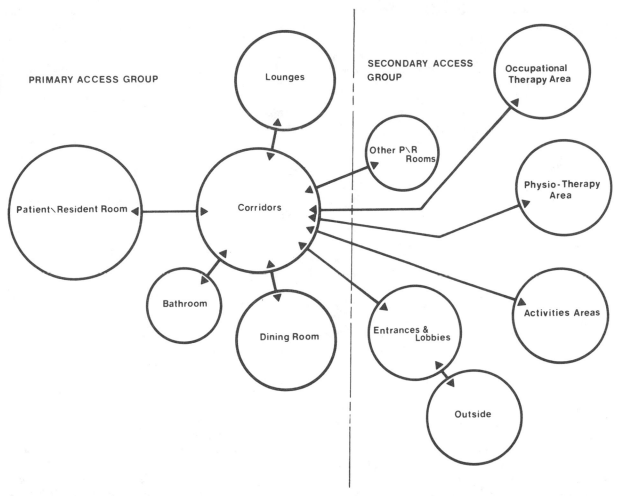

PRIMARY ACCESS GROUP

SECONDARY ACCESS GROUP

Lounges

Occupational Therapy Area

Other P\R Rooms

Physio-Therapy Area

Patient\Resident Room

Corridors

Bathroom

Dining Room

Entrances & Lobbies

Activities Areas

Outside

FIGURE 8

Facility access model. A patient–resident has access to other spaces from his or her own room. In a typical nursing home, therapy and the outside world are essentially removed at least one step from immediate access. This inaccessibility is counterproductive to the rehabilitation process. In an "open"

nursing home, these functions made separate by inaccessibility should be integrated with the primary access group. Therapeutic activities and the outside world should be made tangible parts of primary access, constantly available to the patient–resident.

socialization areas in corridors or in the patient rooms themselves where they would be of potentially more benefit? Thinking in this realm seems to have stagnated for years because of typical architectural solutions and hidebound translations of code from state authorities.

The key to a full realization of the corridor neighborhood and other possibilities for nursing home facilities lies in providing access within the facility. The visitor often tours a facility in just the reverse order of access for the patient-resident. He sees exteriors first, then is shown elaborate lounges, treatment rooms, activity areas, dining rooms, and finally the corridors and rooms. The patient penetrates this same environment from the other direction. He or she resides in a room, has immediate access to the corridor, next the lounge, then the dining room. These penetrations of space are expressed in the accessibility model of Figure 8 (and in Pastalan, 1974).

The accessibility of space to the patient–resident expressed in Figure 8 is depicted graphically by the length and connections of the links. The most inaccessible space to the patient–resident is the outside area of the building and the community. It is complicated to reach by the number of spaces the user must pass through to reach the outside, the connections and distances (links) the user must negotiate, and also by rules and edicts and scrutiny of the staff and administration. The sizes of the spaces are varied to illustrate their various importance in the overall scheme of living of the patient–residents. The corridor assumes, somewhat surprisingly, importance secondary only to the patient–resident room itself. Typically, corridors are thought of as passageways. Codes and regulatory devices are geared to restrict usage to just this function, yet fail to prevent the profound and necessary communications, meetings, and tenor of life the corridor facilitates, abates, and contributes to in the physical environment.

Activity spaces, occupational therapy spaces, and physiotherapy spaces are very nearly the same in importance and access. Various barriers prevent liberal use depending on policies, financial setup of the facility, and administration and staff regulation. Serious questions exist as to whether or not these functions of the facility demand special and physically defined spaces, which are seldom used in a great many facilities. The nature of the physical therapy required in the largest number of nursing homes suggests that devices used for rehabilitation could be built into other areas of the facility as part of an overall concern for use, without the feeling of anxiety promulgated by specialization in this sphere of activity. Ramps, walkways, steps, positioning devices, and other equipment could be built into the more readily usable spaces of the facility, encouraging rehabilitation by its location and the watchfulness and encouragement of the staff. Occupational therapy is so nearly akin to general activity that the two endeavors lend themselves to combination, if not in space allocation then at least in the way they are presented. In fact, much of the general activity found in nursing homes is directly related to occupational therapy even though it may not be prescribed. This also brings to issue whether or not there is nearly enough range and variety in the types of activities available to the aging patient–residents of nursing homes. Many people have hobbies or activities that could easily be integrated with their programs of rehabilitation but are cut out or precluded by a regimented scheme and conception of appropriate activities for this population.

REFERENCES

Baker, Milton J. "Our Society Has Little Use for Anything That's Old." *Ithaca New Times*, June 14, 1973.

Baynes, J. Ronald D. "Environmental Modification for the Older Person." *The Gerontologist*, 11, no. 4 (1971), pt. I.

Koncelik, Joseph A., Edward Ostrander and Lorraine H. Snyder. *The Relationship of the Physical Environment in 6 Extended Care Facilities to the Behavior of Their Resident Aging People.* Research Report No. 103. Ithaca, N.Y.: Cornell University, College of Human Ecology, June 1972.

Morris, Earl, and Margaret E. Woods (eds.). *Housing Crisis and Response: The Place of Mobile Homes in American Life.* Ithaca, N.Y.: Cornell University, College of Human Ecology, June 1972.

Pastalan, Leon A. "Privacy Preferences Among Relocated Institutionalized Elderly." *EDRA 5*, Environmental Research Association, Inc., 1974.

Spivak, Meyer. "Archetypical Place." In *Housing and Environment for the Elderly*, Thomas Byerts (ed.). Washington, D.C.: Gerontological Society, 1973.

BUILDING IN RESIDENCY THROUGHOUT THE FACILITY PLAN

The most essential ingredient, and the one most thoroughly excluded, in present-day nursing homes is providing a sense of residency. There is frequent reference to the "homelike" quality; but this is usually an attempt to provide a visible veneer of appointments and artifacts that relate to the concept of home. However, these attempts are usually found in entrance ways or visitor lounges, and sometimes corridors and other public spaces. These things do not provide a sense of residency because they are not within the control of the patient–resident.

Control over the physical environment by patient–residents depends largely upon five factors:

1. *Mobility status.* Four distinct levels of mobility are found in the nursing home setting: full ambulatory, disabled ambulatory (walk with canes and walkers), semiambulatory (wheelchair bound or geriatric chair bound), and nonambulatory (bedridden). In the semiambulatory category are those who can move their own wheelchairs and those who cannot and are usually seated in geriatric chairs, which cannot be moved by the patient–resident.

2. *Personalization.* The ability of the patient–resident to manipulate artifacts within the physical environment, to bring in personal objects, to affect the character of his or her surroundings in a way that is sympathetic to personal preference.

3. *Socialization.* The ability to commingle with cohorts both in public areas in groups and in privacy, without regulation, threat, or interference.

4. *Privacy.* There must be a place where every patient–resident can go to or retreat to that will permit seclusion for meditation, consultation, intimate discussion, personal activities, and rest. The most logical place for this capability is the patient–resident room, although there may be other conceptions of use of space for this capacity.

5. *Identification.* The patient–resident must feel that he or she belongs in the facility—is not just a recipient—and that the facility belongs to the patient–resident. This can not only be aided through devices in the physical environment itself, but also by including the patient–residents in planning and decision making at the staff and administrative level.

The mobility status of the patient–resident is by far the single most important determining factor in controlling the personal surround and self-maintenance in the overall facility. Mobility status is often the factor used in determining the various segregations of people within the facility by floor or by corridor. Even from the standpoint of staff interest and work load, this seems undesirable. A mix of people may be far more interesting for the staff than people of all similar mobility levels. The problem associated with segregation by any means is that the treatment can be related to a group rather than to the individual. Everyone is handled in the same way. Even superficial scrutiny of policies like this reveals inconsistencies with good residential and health care policy.

The other four factors are largely self-explanatory and will receive further exploration later. However, the key idea is that *choice* should be exercised by the patient–resident in order to have control. Some of the elderly who receive attention do not want control. They are looking for attention—overt, overbearing, and deliberate control of their existence by others. Great care must be exercised at all times by staff so as not to misjudge the desires of patient–residents who require their attention.

If the key is choice and the object is personal control over the environment, including personalization, socialization, identity, and privacy, then residential behavior is being described and defined. In the reports of Snyder et al. (1973) and Koncelik et al. (1973), the essence is observations of existing behaviors with a view toward appropriate changes in nursing homes to provide a foundation for the greatest possible positive behaviors. The second of these reports, available through the College of Human Ecology at Cornell University, is a conference proceedings where specific observations were described and detailed and recommendations were made. Residential behavior relating to health care environments for the aging has largely been developed by Ostrander and Snyder as a concept relating to the physical environment. As social scientists they employ ". . . social science techniques for gathering information in a way that will help [people] understand how spaces and the behavior that takes place within them are related."

The information contained in the two reports mentioned is the basis for the planning information to fol-

low. Owing to the unusual, if not occasionally difficult, combination of design and behavioral science disciplines, the techniques used in generating data in the research projects these reports represent are modifications of existing behavioral science techniques, which permit data collection in such a way as to be more related to the design process. "Behavior mapping" (see Figure 9), for example, was developed to include very refined sets of graphic images to depict behaviors from observations. Over 70 of these "maps" were made during the process of this research. Careful photographic records, many of which are shown in this text, were made to capture various resolutions of current designs and past designs of nursing home spaces. Even more traditional approaches, such as the guided interviews, administrator and staff interviews, and background information, were all devised with a slant toward the physical environment and its relation to its users—both the staff and the patient–residents.

The data pertinent to "residency" or residential behavior refers to four specific spaces in the Koncelik et al. (1973) reports: the bedroom, corridor, lounge, and dining room. These spaces are really the most accessible to the majority of patient–residents in the nursing home, as demonstrated in Figure 8.

FIGURE 9 (*right*)
Index of symbols for behavior maps. The team of researchers who participated in the observation studies of rural nursing homes directed by Koncelik, Ostrander, and Snyder developed this set of visual symbols to be used to express the interactions within the physical environments. Floor plans were drawn prior to the observation studies, and rough maps made on the scene were translated into clear visual images, which successfully demonstrate the richness of activity and potential within these chronic care settings. During the course of the research, 103 behavior mapping records were made. These records included coded records of participants, movement, use of space and objects in space, records of conversations, locations of furnishings, and ambulatory paraphenalia and observer comments. Seventy-two of the mapping studies were translated into visuals, and a sample of these maps is shown in this book through the courtesy of the Department of Design and Environmental Analysis, Cornell University. A special note of gratitude must be extended to Louis Scolnick, who developed the first symbols for the representation of a range of uses.

People

Seated female patient

Seated male patient

Seated aide

Seated nurse

Seated woman

Standing people

Walking people

Observer

Walking Aids

Cane

Walker

Wheelchair

Geriatric Wheelchair

Furniture

Side or dining chair

Side or dining chair w/ arms

Lounge chair

High back chair w/ arms

Geriatric chair

Rocking chair

Captain's chair

Captain's chair w/ arms

Floor or table lamp

Wall lamp

Wastebasket

Assorted end tables

Card or dining table

Over-bed table

T.V., off

T.V., on

Piano

Bed

Activities

Eating

Movement

One-way conversation

Two-way conversation

Undirected conversation

Visual contact

THE BEDROOM

The largest majority of bedrooms found in nursing homes are two-bed arrangements with the beds in parallel. The orientation of the beds places one bed close to the window wall on the exterior and the other near to the closet and doorway. This arrangement usually means that the person in the bed next to the window feels "ownership" of the window and the person located next to the door feels the same about the doorway and closet. This ineffective subdivision of ownership means that one person controls light and ventilation and the other controls visitors, storage, and so on.

The room just described is quite typical, mostly because it is the most expedient solution for a two-bed room conforming to federal and state codes. Any other arrangement will necessitate a greater allocation of space. However, there is a great need to increase the space within the patient–resident room for a variety of reasons, and doing so means that other arrangements are possible. One of the most pressing problems in current arrangements is the lack of ability to move a standard wheelchair around either bed in the two-bed room. Space between walls and bed, furnishings and beds, fixtures and beds, and between beds is insufficient. Current arrangements lead to damage of the space and its furnishings and injury to patients' hands, feet, legs, and arms because of contact with surfaces and edges while moving in wheelchairs and geriatric wheelchairs and during transfers from these devices.

An alternative to the typical two-bed arrangement is to arrange the beds off the centerline of the doorway from the hall with each bed against a wall. In this arrangement, the foot of the bed faces the window with the headboard against a wall (Figure 10). To include the same amenities as the more typical arrangement requires greater space. The arrangement also forces entry during nursing rounds and inspections because the patients are not visible from the hallway. This may be desirable. Entry will usually lead to an exchange of greetings and the opportunity for the patient–residents to express their needs and desires to the staff.

A recommendation that will be explored in greater detail in the design section is that the majority of rooms in nursing homes be *private* rooms. To gain effective control of his or her space, the patient–resident must be the only inhabitant. In single-bed rooms, the occupant can personalize the space, gain privacy, and socialize intimately at his or her discretion without the impedance of another coinhabitant. There will be no effective residential quality when a room is shared. The primary reason for this is that room allocations are the discretion of administration and staff. Rooms are provided on the basis of open bed space and not patient–resident preference. The residents of any given two-bed room may have nothing in common or a great deal in common on the basis of chance. Patient–residents may have physiological or psychological problems that could be mutually detrimental, or, at the least, have unpredictable effects upon each other. Frequently, staff and administrators will report that a coinhabitant of a two-bed room has contracted the physiological or psychological symptoms of the other occupant, even though there was no basis for contagion. In other words, one patient–resident may affect the health status of another by proximity even though neither of the residents has a catching disease. Aside from the marginal chance that two patient–residents will be compatible, the combination of patient–residents in two-bed rooms must be regarded as generally detrimental to rehabilitation, general physiological and mental health, and, of course, the concept of residency.

At the very onset of planning the type of rooms and their interior outfitting, the team engaging in the planning effort must continually be mindful of maximizing the patient–residents' need to personalize the space(s) they inhabit. Obviously, some people will want to make their space a personal expression more than others. However, it is necessary to consider the extreme as the rule. The obvious things brought into nursing home facilities are pictures of the family and small objects that are mementos and stimuli for reminisence. However, personalization extends to wall hangings, pictures of various sizes, large face clocks seen easily from the bed, calendars, bedspreads, chairs, lamps, and so on. As mentioned earlier, a

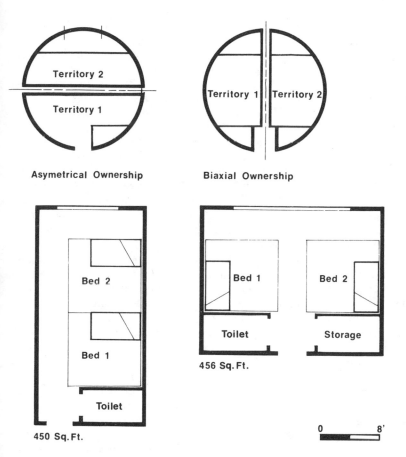

Asymetrical Ownership   Biaxial Ownership

450 Sq. Ft.

456 Sq. Ft.

0   8'

FIGURE 10
Room ownership. In the two-bed room, patient-residents often divide the territory according to the placement of their beds and visual access to the room. "Asymetrical" ownership refers to claims made to different functional parts of the room. "Biaxial" ownership refers to claims made to parts of the room having the same function or the division of a functional part. Patient-residents often control the parts that they claim, which produces friction.

frequently heard report is that some elderly patient-residents bring in the back door from their previous residence and mount it to a wall. This device seems to be a powerful stimulus. The action at a back door over a lifetime is rich and positive.

The room must be designed in such a way as to accommodate a high degree of personalization. Older people in general surround themselves with "clutter." These things are the representative markers of a lifetime. To divest people of these things is to take away very important cues about their ability to control and to seek retaliation. The forms of retaliation used by aging patient-residents are as overt as obstreperous behavior and uncooperativeness and as subtle as pre-

sumed incontinence. What better way to comment about an unsatisfactory environment and irritation about service than to give the staff a problem they dislike intensely and also deface the environment. This is not to suggest that all incontinent patient-residents are protesting through defecation. However, nursing home environments where there is an oppressive custodial atmosphere seem to have the most problems with incontinent patients.

The bathroom attached to the patient-resident room is the only place for privacy for some occupants. However, because of the profound levels of disability found among these populations, very few enter the bathroom unassisted. The healthier patient-resident may use the bathroom as a place for seclusion and meditation. This may also be due to the conflicts found in the two-bed room. Hopefully, privacy can become an integral part of the residential space of the private room, but it will not necessarily follow simply by placing one occupant in a single-bed room. A combination of physical space arrangement and unobtrusive observations by staff must be a fundamental part of the thrust toward privacy for the patient–resident.

CORRIDORS OR HALLWAYS

Because so much activity takes place in corridors, the aging are drawn there either to participate in the activity or to observe it. At the terminus of a hallway, there is an opportunity to sit and watch the activity over quite a distance. The same is true where hallways meet in the nexus of a building. Combine these elements with nursing stations, elevator cores, service areas, and the like, and the attraction is heightened greatly. In the end, the corridor or hallway is the embryonic stage of lounging, and in many ways more attractive because of the potential for passive watching behavior.

Although the corridor is specified as an area of free unencumbered passage, especially from the standpoint of safety and fire hazard, its attractiveness and relationship to neighborhood make it a multifunctional space. To deny that social behavior takes place in the corridor and not provide amenities for this to happen is to double the safety problem and make the hallway increasingly hazardous. For without proper planning in this respect, seating, televisions, eating supports such as adjustable bedstands, and other pieces of equipment find their way into the corridor and encumber the space.

The corridor must be considered a transition space from the patient–resident room in both the social context and in terms of entrance and egress. The "meeting and greeting" going on in the corridor is important and should be facilitated by its design. There have been attempts at an integration of social amenities and mobility. The "therapeutic corridor" designed by a team at the Research and Design Institute in Providence under the direction of Ronald

Beckman is one excellent example of this integration in the corridor of an acute care hospital (Progner, 1971). Similar, if not identical, solutions could be used in nursing home design.

The problems associated with free unencumbered passage are not heightened as a direct result of planning the corridor for interaction and other activity. For the purposes of safety and egress during fire, a free space must remain. Codes and regulations vary on this subject and a width footage is difficult to specify. However, general agreement seems to prevail on an 8-foot unencumbered width. Any alcoves, enclaves, or defined areas of furnishing, which demark the social areas of the corridor, must be outside this free passage area.

The most serious problem associated with passage is the inability of patient–residents to distinguish one area of the corridor from another or one corridor from another. The difficulty involved in institutional corridors is their repetition of elements, sameness, repetitive lighting schemes, low light levels, and glare off highly polished floor surfaces. Combined with excessive corridor length (from the standpoint of perception), repetition of elements provides a very difficult environment to negotiate for a population having sensory deprivation problems. The human sensory system is geared to perceive differences in order to negotiate space. Where there is little difference—in fact, where difference has been unconsciously designed out of an environment—any human sensory system will have difficulty perceiving location and place.

There is, however, the possibility that the concept about socialization space might assist in the creation of cuing about location. Careful demarcations of social areas and lounging areas along the length of a corridor could provide the necessary difference for easy perception of place and location. There should be variation on this theme throughout every corridor so that no length of corridor is the same; they should have their own unique quality and identity.

Free unencumbered passage can also be expedited by careful design of a system of cues. In fact, designers and planners should make every attempt to reinforce signals about locations and place through redundant cuing. It is possible that visual, auditory, and textural cues can be carefully implanted to tell people where they are. Various possibilities for cuing mechanisms will be explored in Part IV.

LOUNGES

In the current state of the art of building of nursing homes, lounges must be regarded as the single greatest failure as a concept. Typical lounges are the result of regulations which specify that so many square feet must be devoted to lounge space on the basis of number of beds. This device usually results in one or more very large areas devoted to socialization, relaxation, and contemplation, but not really accommodating any of these activities.

Lorraine Snyder and her coworkers (1973) offers a perception on the problems of lounges: "It is as though the designer has said, 'Here, eating will take place; here social activity will take place.' We found that people do not compartmentalize activities, particularly when [two] are taking place at the same time."

This reflection points up one of the serious difficulties with present lounges: they are multifunctional, but so designed and planned as to be inhibiting to the behaviors they were meant to support. The large open space that usually characterizes the lounge is counterproductive to intimate communications between two people or small groups. Many activities will be taking place at the same time, and because of the rigid scheduling of activities in homes for the aging, very little activity will take place at other times. In fact, the observations of the team under Koncelik, Ostrander, and Snyder (1972) show that a great many lounges were totally unoccupied for extended periods of the day.

Another important consideration is the furnishing of the lounge space. In extended care facilities, between 30 and 70 percent of the population was confined to wheelchairs. Yet, the majority of lounges are furnished as if everyone residing in the nursing home was ambulatory. These furnishings are usually encumbrances and impediments to free access in the lounge to desirable space. To accommodate the greater share of patient–residents in most nursing homes, sensitive staff members will shove unused furnishings out of the way or relocate them in some other place to allow free access. This solution is not totally satisfactory, because if the furniture remains in the lounge portions, the space becomes unsuitable for use and unaccessible.

Another related factor involved with groupings and activities is that a great many patient–residents who use the lounge are transported there by staff members. The location of people in the lounge may be at the discretion of the staff and not the patient–residents. This can explain clusters of users jammed near a doorway in the lounge or lined up very precisely at a window. While it is difficult to socialize when side by side with another person, this linear configuration is often found in lounges, entranceways, and lobbies. It is also a function of the maintenance environment.

The staff who care for the facility are often the people who determine the alignment of furnishings and conversational groupings. It is easier to push a broom or a mop through a space if the chairs are out of the way against a wall then if they are in clusters in the middle of the room. Thus even the ambulatory patient–residents are forced to use space and furnishings at the discretion of staff on occasion.

Lounges can either be isolated and enclosed, with access through a doorway or passageway, or they can be open areas near an entrance, at the intersection of hallways, or in a space not unlike a harbor just off a corridor to one side or both sides. Either of these solutions has its own set of problems, which must be ameliorated if successful social behavior is to take place. The isolated lounge is less attractive than the open lounge because there is less potential for activity that can be passively observed. The open lounge provides access to high activity levels for passive observation, but it does not permit effective interchange among the occupants of the space. There is so much going on that it interferes with discussion, intimate communications, and activities that need a degree of isolation to be fully effective.

The need for fresh design approaches to lounges in new facilities and some modifications in existing nursing homes is obvious. As they stand, lounges are not fulfilling their intended role adequately—nor any other role ascribed to them. Lounges need to be *smaller* and more accessible to the whole population within the nursing home setting. *This means transferring space devoted to lounges to patient–resident rooms.* It also means utilizing lounge space in corridors for transitional social spaces. In truth, it means abandoning the well-worn concept of an isolated multifunctional room, which does nothing well and is a very great waste of money.

DINING ROOMS

It is fair to say that meals are the most highly anticipated activity of the day in nursing homes. They offer an opportunity to divest the mind of thoughts about sickness and decreasing lack of capability and to think about and talk about something external to problems of self. Some nursing home staffs go to great lengths to make meals an event and to encourage the participation of the aging in their care in a social as well as nutritional activity. Yet, dining rooms are underutilized in many nursing homes. In some facilities, sometimes 50 percent or fewer of the patient–residents take their meals in the dining room. There are two reasons for this: (1) a substantial proportion of the population cannot go to the dining room and must be provided meals in their rooms; (2) a number of residents will not go to the dining room because of their embarrassment over appearance, inability to eat without assistance, or the condition of the space itself. Dining rooms can be very noisy, and, as stated in the section on the physiology of aging, conversation becomes indistinguishable from background noise for many of the elderly.

Once in the dining room, a very apparent problem inhibits access. Dining rooms seem to be designed from the standpoint of seating as many patient–residents as possible without fully considering the effect upon passage, serving of food, and the ability to penetrate beneath table surfaces and egress backward from this position.

A noted nursing home completed in 1972 in New York City opened a dining room in a nursing wing accommodating the planned population of that wing in two sittings. Because of the large number of wheelchairs used, the free passage was insufficient. Problems arose very quickly when the last few to be seated could not be maneuvered into any table area. Jams

occurred. The staff became quickly frustrated. As a result, tables were removed, existing furnishings were rearranged, and the meals were served in three sittings. This, of course, increased costs because of extending staff time, reduced the quality of service and food, and discouraged the patient–residents from using the facility.

Other homes have found that tables purchased did not permit penetration of wheelchairs or the large geriatric wheelchairs beneath the apron of the table. This meant that the distance from the table to the person was so great that transfer of food was very difficult, even without lack in motor control or arthritis. Eating under these conditions was embarrassing and difficult. Few patient–residents will tolerate these conditions for very long. Finally, as observed in the course of research by the Koncelik, Ostrander, and Snyder teams (Snyder et al., 1973), patient–residents drifted away from using the dining room in one facility and all meals were delivered to rooms.

Other problems that seem minor at first are serious detriments to full utilization of dining facilities. Chairs for the ambulatory elderly should have arms. When chairs do have arms, they too must be able to penetrate beneath the apron of the table. It is not uncommon to observe dining chairs with arms in nursing homes that will not penetrate beneath the apron of the dining table.

Table selection is also an important factor and one that has received a great deal of attention. The number of people in a grouping, the size of table in relation to both entrance and egress and also serving, and the configuration—round, square, rectilinear or ovaloid—receive as much discussion as the table shape for a summit meeting. However, the table selected for a nursing home is probably more important in many ways. The four-position table provides a configuration that places everyone in view of one another. A round table allows approach by a staff member from any side for serving and no discriminatory seating positions. However, others argue that because of the high degree of socialization that should be taking place in the dining room, a six- or eight-position table is better. It is axiomatic that the larger the table the more problems there will be in terms of entrance, egress, and service. Large banquet-type tables are not desirable for the nursing home dining room. The side-by-side eating position is not at all conducive to conversation and promotes crowding and impedes ease of eating.

Although the dining room is, at this juncture, a more successful space generally than the lounge, it has succeeded because it has a definite function and can be made attractive because of the high degree of activity. However, not all eating or feeding takes place in the dining room. Patient-residents eat in lounges, hallways, bedrooms, outside, and elsewhere. Although the meal is a spur to interaction, large conglomerations of people and equipment to handle the service of food in one place detract from the meal and irritate the patient-residents with hearing impediments. Dining rooms should be *smaller* and more intimate, using small tables conducive to conversation. It is also possible that some patient-residents who have problems eating, but use the dining facility, need something of a semiprivate area for their meals.

With the realization that all eating and feeding does not take place in the dining room, it should be recognized that dining facilities can be provided elsewhere; perhaps they should be included as part of a "therapeutic" corridor or part of the patient-resident room. The important factor is to recognize that, in spite of regulatory devices, the eating or feeding function takes place as much outside the dining room and therefore should be accommodated elsewhere if the facility is to be totally effective.

To summarize the discussion of social behavior within a nursing home facility and the concept of "residency," it is clear that the primary group of archetypical spaces plays the greatest role in effective provision of these important precepts of the open concept of design. The patient-resident must feel that he or she has some measure of control over the physical environment he or she comes in contact with. This is accomplished through personalizing private spaces and attaining privacy and intimacy in the patient-resident room and elsewhere. It is accomplished by removing physical and psychological barriers to free access and full utilization of the environment. Moreover, control and residency can only be accomplished when there is a realization of the real uses of space and the range of behaviors the patient-residents exhibit, and a balance is struck between the distribution of health care services and the residential quality of a facility.

REFERENCES

Koncelik, Joseph A., Edward Ostrander, and Lorraine H. Snyder. *The Relationship of the Physical Environment in 6 Extended Care Facilities to the Behavior of Their Resident Aging People.* Research Report No. 103. Ithaca, N.Y.: Cornell University, College of Human Ecology, June 1972.

Progner, Jean. "The Sociologist and the Designer Can Be Friends." *Design and Environment*, New York, 1971 (see p. 147).

Snyder, Lorraine, E. Ostrander, and J. A. Koncelik. *The New Nursing Home.* Conference Proceedings. Ithaca, N.Y.: Cornell University, College of Human Ecology, 1973.

DESIGN AND OUTFITTING OF PATIENT-RESIDENT ACCESSIBLE SPACES

The premise of this text is that rehabilitation and "openness" in the design of a nursing home facility are dependent upon the conformation of residential areas within the facility and the emphasis of residency as a quality throughout the facility. The physical environment should impart to the patient-resident a feeling of control: control over the patient-resident's own person and destiny and control over his or her immediate surroundings. This means designing the physical plant so that users who have physical and psychological deficits can negotiate within it, determine their own actions to the highest degree possible, and manipulate various components within the setting that are ordinarily left to staff but provide a sense of self-reliance to the aging patient-resident.

This capsulization of intent and direction is the essential ingredient in moving toward greater openness in nursing home design. It should be recognized that these facilities are not just health care operations but places where people live for a substantial length of time. However, it is indeed as important to recognize that attitudes and methods of health care delivery must change to accommodate openness along with design.

The first, and most important, recommendation is to reduce the size of public spaces or large open and isolated lounges, and to move a substantial portion of the square footage delegated to these spaces into resident rooms and a new concept of corridor neighborhood. An alternative to this approach is to increase the size of private rooms and employ therapeutic or social corridors, and leave the other spaces at present levels of space requirements. However, this serves no purpose at all. The alternative approach increases the cost of the facility substantially, retains the outdated concepts of residency, which are wasteful and not effective, and provides an even more confusing environment to the user with even less accessibility.

There must be a full commitment to the concept if it is to be employed at all. In this way, the facility may be condensed in size, space allocations are shifted, not increased, and the total impact of the physical plant should be increased for the better.

In essence, this shift in spatial allocation means an increase in square footage in the patient-resident room and *the building of a large majority of single patient-resident rooms*. At least 80 percent of the patient-resident rooms should be private rooms.

The "corridor neighborhood," described by the

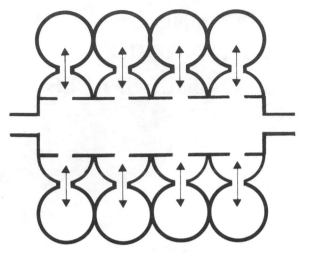

**Lounge Space Redistributed as
Social Space Outside Rooms**

FIGURE 11
Possible corridor scheme. To achieve a "corridor neighborhood" lounge spaces should be distributed differently in association with the room entrances. These smaller "free access" social spaces would act as the front porch of each room. A greater variety of visual stimuli would be an inherent part of this type of arrangement, lessening the confusion of patients due to the repetitious character of typical corridor configurations.

Presseys' in Part II, receives the most radical change in design from that of the unifunctional designs of corridors and hallways in previous facilities. Isolated space delegated to activity rooms, physiotherapy, occupational therapy, and to some degree dining space should be integrated with the space in the corridor neighborhood. Lounges should become alcove- or bay-type spaces off high-activity locations of corridors, and dining spaces should become smaller, more intimate spaces, segregated from the corridors but placed within each wing of any given facility (see Figures 11, 12, and 13).

PATIENT–RESIDENT ROOM

The square footage requirement for private patient–resident rooms should increase to 180 square feet, designated by a rectilinear form 12 feet wide by 15 feet long. The bathroom area, including a minimum of lavatory and toilet, should be isolated from this space. A residential or social area should be provided and visually separated from the bed area, but falling within the 180 square feet demarcated outside the bathroom space. There are five distinct components of the patient–resident room (Figure 14). They are as follows.

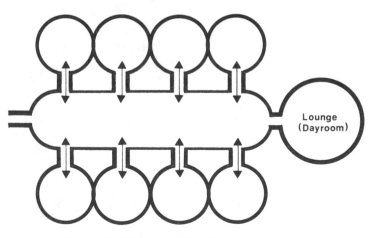

Typical Double-Loaded Corridor

FIGURE 12
Typical corridor scheme. Often regarded as efficient, especially in high-rise construction, the double-loaded corridor presents acute sensory problems for the aging infirm. The repetitiousness and similarity of elements contribute to confusion and the tunnel-like quality of most long corridors greatly contributes to the overall institutional quality of nursing homes. Lounges at the end of corridors have been shown by several researchers to be ineffective social spaces or activity spaces owing to the lack of potential for passive engagement in watching.

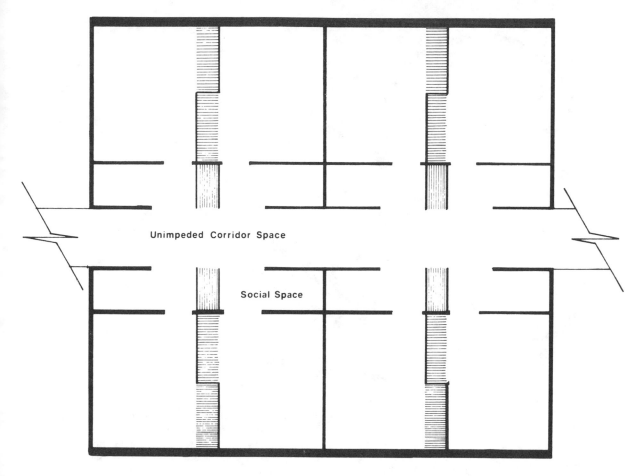

Back-to-Back Room Configuration

FIGURE 13

Corridor neighborhood with private rooms. There is a greater possibility for unimpeded traffic flow where there is integral, free-access social space. Many nursing homes suffer from clogged halls because they function as meeting and therapy areas in spite of the codes and their lack of amenities.

Resting-Sleeping Area

This space includes the bed and is also a space from which the patient–resident can control the rest of the room. The bed itself requires a great deal more design attention than it has received (Parsons, 1972), but should definitely not be a standard hospital bed. It should be wider than those presently found in nursing homes and lower. It should accommodate resting, sitting, and sleeping behaviors. The bed should be conducive to sexual behavior or easily adjustable or movable to accommodate a second bed for sexual activity. Sexual activity takes place in nursing homes between husbands and wives and partners who make acquaintance and form unions in the nursing home as patient-residents (Figure 15).

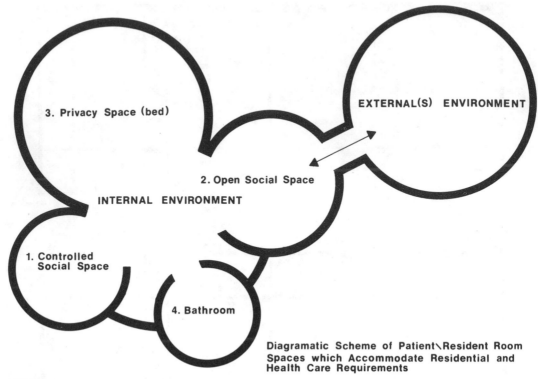

Diagramatic Scheme of Patient\Resident Room Spaces which Accommodate Residential and Health Care Requirements

FIGURE 14

Patient-resident room scheme. A truly effective room for a nursing home patient must be *residential* as well as medical–nursing in design character. To achieve this quality, privacy and socialization must be controlled by the patient-resident. Private rooms should constitute the majority of living arrangements. Two-bed rooms, preferably designed for biaxial territoriality, should only be used for bedfast patients receiving the greatest possible medical attention within the constraints of nursing home care.

The bed should also be personalizable, with top coverings brought in by the patient–residents if they so desire. This is a primary area where individuality can be exercised, especially for the bedridden.

There should be *4 feet* of clearance between the bed and all other objects and walls for penetration by the wheelchair if access is desirable or suggested by an opening. Three feet is not sufficient to permit proper penetration, especially when the hands of a patient-resident are included on the outside of the wheels of the chair (Figure 16).

Placement of the bed with respect to natural lighting from windows is very important in the control of glare. There should be sufficient flexibility for bed location so that the patient–resident can adjust or reposition the bed according to personal preference.

A most neglected area of concern is accident prevention around the bed and reduction of injuries because of falls near the bed. A recent study conducted by Richard Kieselbach and Richard Hatch under the supervision of Joseph Koncelik (1975) at the Ohio State University in conjunction with a leading retirement community showed that the largest majority of falls and injuries due to falls occur around the bed—not the bathroom. Fully 60 percent of all reported injuries in the facility occurred near the bed. Injuries

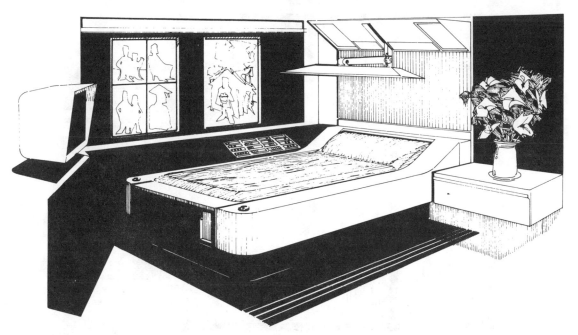

FIGURE 15

Within the area surrounding the bed, there should be visual access to controls for light, heating and cooling, tele-vision and radio, nurse call, and also some degree of personalization. The control units often mounted behind the bed for the convenience of staff should be mounted at bed level within easy reach, as shown in the illustration. The bed itself should be wider and equipped with rolled soft bolsters that would allow sitting for dressing and visiting. The bolsters should also allow for the mounting of a canopy or oxygen tent.

were substantial because of contact with sharp edges and corners of the furnishings around this area of the living space. It was often found that water accumulat-ing on the floor of the bathroom would spill into the bedroom area and cause injury or fall after bathing or other activity in the bath or elsewhere in the facility. The ramifications for bed design are that the structural elements should be designed with rounded or "softened" corners, and the area around the bed should have a surface that would provide stability when wet (Figure 15).

Even though the bathroom is potentially dangerous, the activity in the bath is largely assisted by staff. Ac-cidents are frequently avoided in the bathroom be-cause someone is there to help.

The various additional functions of the nursing home bed need intensive study at this point. This specifically refers to those health care functions which largely determine the hospital bed. The degree to which all the hospital functions (trandelenberg, reverse trandel-enberg, etc.) are needed in this equipment is not clear. One obvious impediment for staff and patients is the bed rail. Although there are occasions where restraint is necessary, the rails in the down position are dan-gerous and a barrier to easy entrance and egress from the bed. Nurses report that they bruise their shins from making beds and patients have become entangled or slipped on them when egressing from the bed (Figure 20).

Figures 15 through 20 illustrate some problems and solutions in relation to bed placement and use.

There is enough information and informed opinion to justify study and design development of a nursing home bed—separate in conception and product type

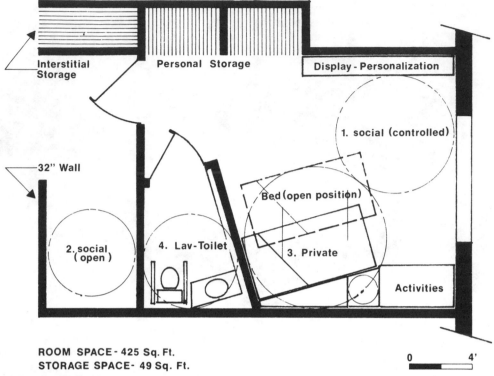

ROOM SPACE - 425 Sq. Ft.
STORAGE SPACE - 49 Sq. Ft.

FIGURE 16

There are many possible configurations for the private room. However, they should all include consideration of the functional attributes depicted in Figure 14. This plan is an attempt to "make real" some of the considerations, such as display for personalization, visual access from the bed, and storage. "Interstitial" storage refers to connective storage between rooms, which would be used for unused wheelchairs, furnishings, and seasonal clothing.

from the hospital bed. It is also possible that more than one type of bed should be available in the nursing home to accommodate changing needs and the range of requirements exhibited by the resident population.

Social–Activity Area

A space should be set aside within the patient–resident room and isolated to some degree to be used for private conversations with friends and relatives, cohorts and acquaintances from the facility, and others; private use for reading, sleeping, thinking; and personal activities—knitting, sewing, model building,

writing, painting, sculpting, and so on. This space should be furnished so that it can be adjusted or rearranged to suit various purposes. Furniture should be removed at the request of the patient–resident (Figure 14).

The minimum furniture required for this space is two lounge chairs with arms and foot rests, a 30-inch high table suitable for four residents to be seated at (with optional folding chairs or side chairs; see reference to furnishings on pages 135–137), and a glare-reduced or balanced reading lamp (Figure 21).

There are a variety of methods for isolating areas within a total space. It is not always necessary to use

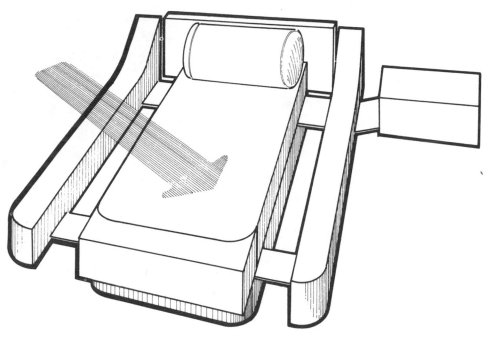

FIGURE 17
The bed used in nursing homes should be wider than a hospital bed and should not have rails, as a general rule. Rails may be mounted when restraint is required for medical reasons. Greater width allows for more freedom of movement during sleep and for sexual relations. In the open position, the bolsters should move away allowing access for changing the bedding or allowing a double-wide mattress for more suitable accommodation of conjugal visits.

walls to locate single elements or groupings of furnishings. Lighting, both artificial and natural, can be the medium through which isolation is achieved. The orientation of the bed to other furnishings is another way in this particular case. Or partial walls, planters, partitions, hangings, or sculpted panels could be used for decorative effect, isolation, and then removed if not desired by the party occupying the space.

This particular area, the patient–resident room, must be regarded as needing the most essential changes in the total concept of the nursing home. Trends at present seem to be gravitating toward greater controlled environments and away from residential quality. Research is showing that these sterile and autocratic environments fill the aging who must reside in them

with anxiety. It is misleading to suggest that withdrawal is symptomatic of old age. It is far more accurate to report that withdrawal is a consequence of not being able to retain attachments and control. In other words, it is difficult to use the term withdrawal as a representative classification for a malady when it is the surround, both social and physical, that has withdrawn from the afflicted. It is like throwing a man into the Hudson River with cement overshoes and then claiming he drowned because he could not swim strongly enough to overcome his personal deficits.

Maintaining a social–activity area in the personal space of the patient–resident is a way of retaining the much needed attachments to life before institutionalization. Even if the space is not used directly or with conscious purpose, because it is there, it can be

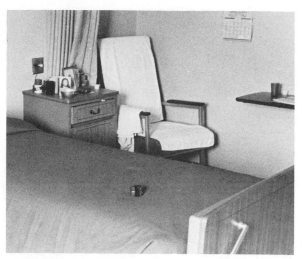

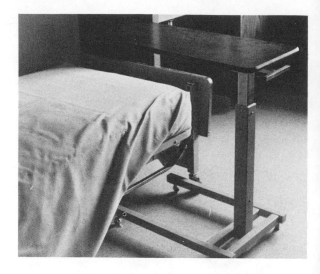

FIGURE 18

Bed "surround" in a typical nursing home. Objects that surround the bed are not carefully considered in terms of their relationship to the bed and each other. As the area of privacy, there should be means of controlling the room and objects from the bed (at least in terms of placement preference, if not actual change or modulation). The traditional feeding table, as an example, is designed to be operated by the staff, not by the patient–resident. (Photo: John Kelsey and Robert Steinbugler.)

seen, or used by friends and relatives to provide a residence in control of the patient–resident.

Recently, codes designed in various states are requiring that lavatories be moved into the living space of the patient–resident room. The exact reasons for this change are unclear. One reason given is that it is for the convenience of the staff who wash up outside the bathroom after attending or before attending the patient–resident. Another part of this explanation is that staff members are often tempted to clean bedpans in the room of the patient rather than carry them to the sterilizer usually placed somewhere else on the wing or in the building. Moving the lavatory outside the bathroom with the toilet makes it difficult for the staff member to shortcut this operation. However, it is unfortunate that the patient–resident must pay a high penalty for the lack of consideration—and sometimes training—of others. This kind of change in the physical environment is one more example of a loss of control and superinstitutionalization of the environment. There are probably a multitude of ways whereby the problem of an unwanted job can be accomplished without ensuring against a health hazard at the expense of the very people the facility is supposed to serve.

The flexibility of this area is most important. The patient–resident should be able to exert maximum control over the number of furnishings in this space, make changes from time to time, and arrange the chosen objects at his or her discretion and preferred location.

It is important to exclude furnishings from use in nursing home facilities that have been shown to have a detrimental effect on the users' abilities and upon socialization. A 30-inch-high table is recommended for the social-activity area in the patient–resident room and any other area where socialization is to be encouraged. Low coffee tables, frequently found in many public spaces outside the nursing home and in nursing homes, are too low to suffice as effective "magnets" for the elderly infirm to gather around. Low tables allow the various participants in conversational groupings to see the least functional part of the body, the legs. The 30-inch-high table forces

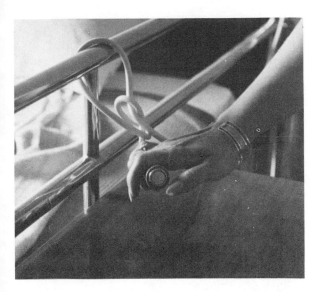

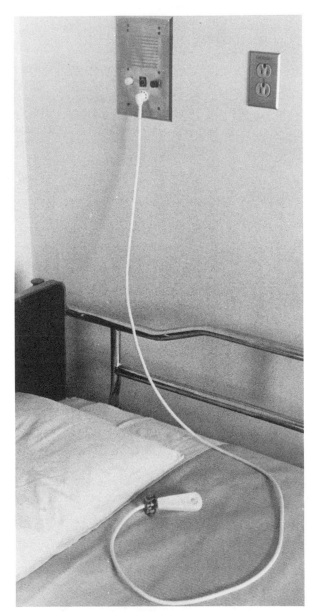

FIGURE 19
Bed surround controls. The inaccessibility of nurse call buttons on walls either above or behind the reach of the patient–resident is not helped by long extension cords, which become entangled in the bedding or pulled out of the wall socket. (Photo: John Kelsey and Robert Steinbugler.)

visual concentration upon the most functional part of the body.

Snyder et al. (1973) commented that, if a 30-inch-high table were to be moved near a window in a lounge, the view to the outside plus the effect of the table "masking" the lower portion of the body might be an effective method of increasing the socialization in public spaces. Experiments have been carried out whereby a 30-inch-high table was placed in a lounge area, and it was observed that groupings did form

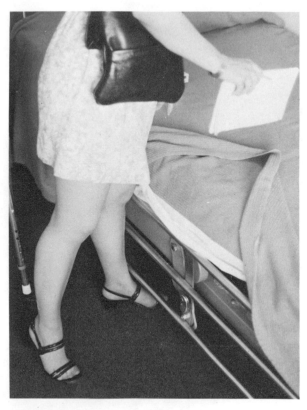 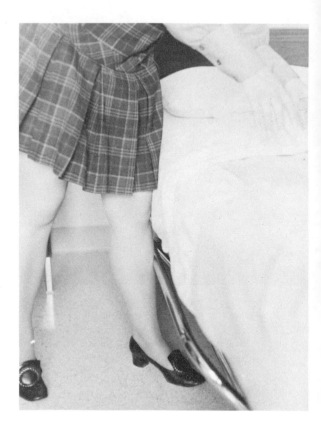

FIGURE 20
Bed rail. Lowered bed rails are dangerous to the ambulatory patient-resident and are an obstruction to efficient bed making by staff. Accidents often occur when feet become entangled in the rail while getting out of bed or when the rail drops when it has not been properly secured. (Photo: John Kelsey and Robert Steinbugler.)

Display Space

One of the most important facets in providing a measure of control, as stated previously, is providing the opportunity to personalize the space the patient-resident inhabits. Display space cannot be isolated in the manner of the bed space or the social-activity area. Display is going on, either in a deliberate way or indeliberate way, everywhere in the room. Remove all stimuli from the room and there is actually a negative display going on, a display that communicates a powerful message to those infirm about where they are and what is happening to them.

There should be absolutely minimal restrictions on the hanging of pictures, calendars, fabric hangings, and other accoutrements. Strip mouldings are available that allow for this type of personalization without damage to the walls. Shelving units should be provided so that books, photos in display stands, memorabilia, and other personal articles can be stored and seen (Figure 21).

It is probably more appropriate to locate the greater

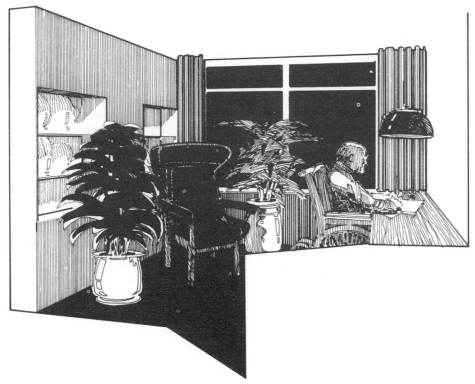

FIGURE 21
Residential quality depends upon having "living room" space under the control of the patient. The
space should accommodate either two lounge chairs or one lounge chair and a wheelchair.

share of shelving for display in the socialization–
activity area and the devices for picture hanging in
the area where they can be seen from the bed. It is
important to note that many patient-resident rooms
presently in use do not provide any means for display
so that personal effects can be seen from the bed.
The view from the bed is extremely important. Divest
this surround of meaning and richness and delay or
subvert rehabilitation.

A greatly overlooked area, which could be a source
of rich communications in a very subtle way, is the
ceiling of the patient-resident room. For the bedridden or those very incapacitated, the ceiling becomes
a dominant part of the physical environment, especially from the bed. This is not to suggest that each
room should become a miniature Sistine Chapel, al-

though the relationship is quite clear. Textured surfaces, subtle gradients of paint, patterns, and other
devices could be used as intriguing reliefs on a surface
that is little attended to as an important source of
visual stimulation. Other cultures use regular geometric
patterns or spirals as a visual cue for contemplation.
The patterns need not be excessive and should be a
reflection of the overall interior design of the room.
This kind of surface treatment could also be a locating
device, marking the approximate distance away for
the room occupant or bed occupant. A white ceiling
can seem to be an endless depth.

Another possibility that should not be overlooked
is the use of the ceiling for hanging draped materials,
colorful pictures, photographs, even the American
flag. Careful and judicious placement and choices

could also visually isolate areas. For instance, the bed or sleeping–resting area could be effectively isolated by draped materials that are also fixed to the ceiling.

Storage Space

The designation of display separate from storage is a deliberate one. Things that the patient–resident displays are in view for a variety of reasons; cuing the room occupant about reminisences, well-being, and control are some of them. Those things to be stored are not to be viewed, but their future use requires ready access. Among these items may be clothing, personal objects and products, nonperishable foods, writing materials, cosmetics, brushes and combs, etc. (Figures 13 and 16).

It is important for the patient–resident to retain the maximum amount of clothing and personal effects possible. Frequently, prolonged stay in a nursing home means progressive loss of personal effects, a powerful signal about one's own status. The problem is that facilities rarely plan or possess adequate storage or an efficient means of retrieving stored goods for their occupants. There should be three kinds of storage available to the occupant of a patient–resident room: drawer-type storage and cabinet storage for personal effects used daily and previous possessions, closet storage for clothing in season and larger items, and dead storage outside the space for personal effects and furniture used only occasionally or periodically.

This last type of storage could be located in space adjoining the patient–resident room or in central cores in wings with double corridors. This storage space is not to be confused with the type of permanent storage the facility staff might need for their own use. The patient–resident should have access to this space to survey his or her possessions or available furnishings for changes in the room. Access to the space should be from outside the patient–resident room so that staff can assist in use and making choices (Figure 16).

The Bathroom

There should be an isolated space containing a lavatory with mirror and storage, a toilet, and bath with shower. This space should be sufficiently large to allow penetration and withdrawal of a wheelchair from the area surrounding each of the three installed fixtures mentioned. In addition, since a great many patient–residents will be assisted in the bathroom area, there should be room for maneuvering for both parties and the ambulatory aid (Figure 22).

Generally speaking, lavatories are mounted too high. The sink bowls chosen are too deep to allow penetration by the wheelchair and then easy use of the fixture. Faucets and activators on sinks should be side mounted to expedite ease of reach and use, and the activators clearly marked or color-coded to assure proper direction for the desired temperature of water. The surfaces on the sink may be very slippery when they are wet, which reduces the ability of the patient-resident to grasp controls or articles on the surface adjoining the sink itself. Control knobs could be oversized and textured for identification as well as ease of grasp (Figure 22).

The mirror above the sink is given little attention in most current architecture in nursing homes. It is usually mounted too high and acts as the cover of a storage case in the same manner of most residential construction. This is almost a totally unworkable solution for the majority of those who must use this item. The mirror should be mounted as close to the level of the sink as possible, perhaps just above the backsplash of the lavatory console, or as an integrated part of the lavatory console. Another improvement that has been tried successfully in some nursing homes is to cant the mirror outward at the top. This will provide a viewing surface that even the smallest lady in a wheelchair will be able to use (Figure 23).

There must be new solutions sought for the bathroom storage problem. Storage behind the mirror is totally inadequate as a design solution for the wheelchair user. Storage could be integrated into the console of the lavatory—both open storage for ready access to washcloths, soap, toothbrushes, and the like, and closed storage for bottles, tubes, jars, and other paraphernalia likely to be used for personal toiletry (Figure 22).

The toilet presents problems that are in some cases resolvable and in other cases very difficult to resolve. There is no conclusive information on the height at which a toilet should be mounted to expedite its use

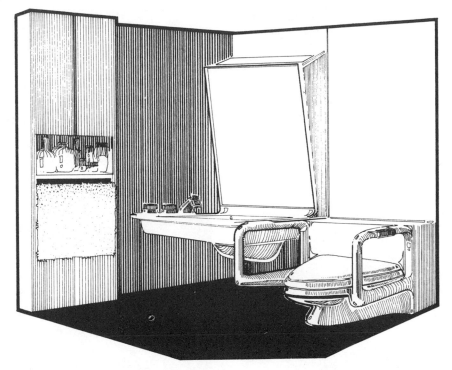

FIGURE 22
The bathroom. There should be sufficient space to move about, especially in a wheel-chair, in the bathroom for transfers and grooming. Transfers require handrails on *both* sides of the toilet because there is a high frequency of paralysis or reduced strength on one side in most nursing home populations. The sink area should have accessible, clearly marked controls, and the mirror to the rear of the sink should be canted for the wheel-chair user. Storage, quite lacking in most institutional bathrooms, should be sufficient to accommodate the grooming needs of the user.

and ease waste excretion from the human body. Kira's *The Bathroom* (1966) poses some interesting concepts for all the units or fixtures in the bathroom, but the height of the toilet from the floor is questionable. A low toilet would help in the excreting function, but have a detrimental effect upon the ability of the elderly to get on and off. Many toilets in nursing homes are equipped with devices that raise the seat, or the toilets are higher to start with.

One serious problem that can be resolved is the use of grab bars around the toilet. Frequently, only one grab bar is mounted to a wall while the other side of

the toilet has none. Many of the elderly patient-residents have use of only one side of their body. Hopefully, in nursing homes where the grab bar is on the right side, the largest majority are fully functional on that side. There should be bars on both sides of the toilet and they should be as close in to the top surface as possible. The maximum amount of force anyone is able to exert with the hands and arms is straight downward. If an elderly person has to reach out forward and grab one or two assist bars, he or she will be helped less than if he or she can exert thrust directly downward. Bars in this position will be less

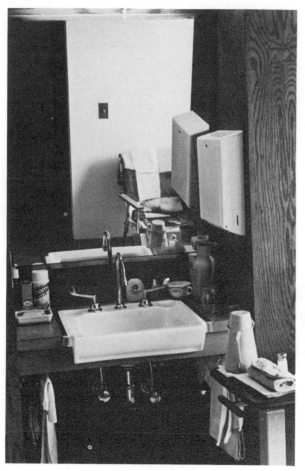

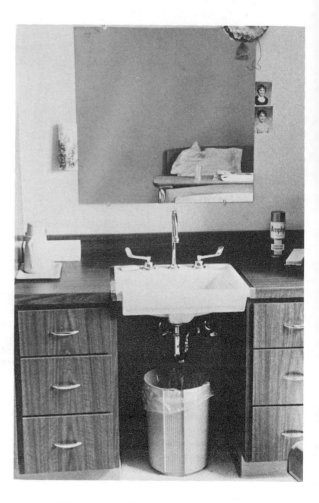

FIGURE 23

Lavatory "center." Today, lavatories are often designed to fit in the controlled social space of the patient–resident room, an inappropriate location. This arrangement, for whatever reasons, nullifies residential atmosphere in the room setting. However, the basic concept of a washing and grooming area specially designed for wheelchair users is essential, and the shallow draft sink and canted mirror arrangement shown in the left photo provide a more usable configuration. (Photo: John Kelsey and Robert Steinbugler.)

of an impediment to the wheelchair getting close in to the toilet as well (Figure 22).

In many instances where space is a premium, the lavatory console is used as a secondary support along with the grab rail on the wall or mounted to the floor. Unfortunately, the lavatory top surface is often wet and slippery with no traction or surface to grasp for purchase. This is not a recommended way to have patient-residents lift themselves from the toilet.

The flushing mechanism should be easily found, identified, and used. Many flushing mechanisms are placed in the most difficult areas to reach while seated on the toilet. It is possible that a specialized toilet should be developed which incorporates support rails, positioning saddle, and forward-mounted flushing mechanism. Although a device of this type would initially benefit the nursing home patient-resident, it has potential in other commercial and residential construction projects as well.

Lighting

Special mention must be given to one other facet of patient-resident room design because of its overall importance and some recent findings, which have a great deal of bearing upon perception of the room and its use.

Lighting, both natural and artificial, must be considered very carefully and manipulated thoughtfully. Most patient-resident rooms are accessible from a double-loaded corridor. The lighting in the corridor is usually low if not insufficient to begin with. When the patient-resident enters his or her room, there is immediate confrontation with a window wall on the far side of the room and during the day, high glare. It will take the elderly patient-resident some time to adapt to this light, and even after adaptation there will be insufficient discrimination of fine details or objects. This is a moment in time when there is a great deal of potential for accident and injury.

A possible remedy for this problem is to have an entrance area from the corridor in which the light level is higher, but not as contrasted as it now is. Another possibility is to baffle the light entering the room through a screen or shutters on the outside of the window wall. There are an infinite variety of solutions to this problem, but they remain to be sought because the basic problem has gone unrecognized.

Another key lighting factor that also bears closer attention is the difference in quantities of light entering the eye of a standing person as opposed to a seated person in the overall facility. Kieselbach and Hatch's report (1975) documents the results from lighting level studies conducted in one facility in daylight and artificial light conditions. In almost every area of the facility, the quantities of light were *different* for the walking ambulatory eye height measure and the wheelchair seated eye height. Astoundingly, some surfaces receiving the same light—both quantitatively and qualitatively—gave different reflected readings for the two positions (Figure 24).

At the lower eye height, there is more direct exposure to shrouded bulbs, which are unexposed to the eye of an ambulatory person. However, signs, general area lighting from the ceiling, and indirect lighting are at levels determined for the ambulatory person.

It should become policy in nursing homes to check lighting levels from two positions. As stated previously, somewhere between 30 and 80 percent of the patient-residents are nonambulatory or semiambulatory in wheelchairs or geriatric chairs. Lighting should be planned and designed into a facility to accommodate both the ambulatory and wheelchair eye height positions.

In general, there should be greater use of indirect lighting and greater use of balanced lighting sources—combinations of incandescent and fluorescent lighting sources to reduce glare. Because of the wide use of hard flooring surfaces and the commensurate problem of high gloss when cleaned, there should be greater use of peripheral lighting in rooms and corridors. Identification panels in rooms and corridors might be backlighted transluscent panels.

Lighting could also be far more carefully chosen to flatter the people who occupy the facility. Much of the present lighting creates harsh shadows that distort features and overemphasize health problems. Even staff will suffer in this respect. Fluorescent lighting flatters no one when it is used by itself. Only if a given facility is willing to spend additional monies on better-quality fluorescents will there be an adequate lighting scheme to compliment the facility and its people.

THE CORRIDOR NEIGHBORHOOD

The concept exemplified by the change from the traditional treatment of the corridor is a recognition that the rooms are residences and the corridor is an avenue on which people live. In this sense, patient-residents should find their activities, recreation therapy, and friends close to home territory. Like an avenue, the corridor should allow for the same identification of specific places where individuals live.

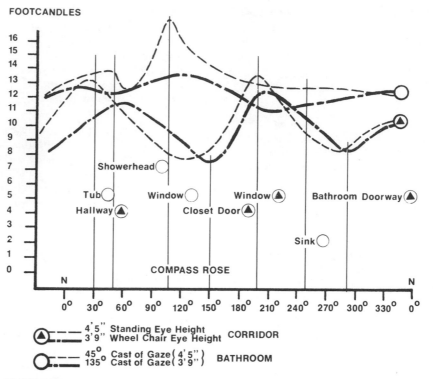

FOOTCANDLES

FIGURE 24

Diagram of perceptible illumination. Illumination seen by the occupant of a space and measurements of general illumination are two distinctly different things. This diagram illustrates that illumination (and consequent glare) flucuate in any given space, and that perception is different in the same location for the wheelchair user and the ambulatory user. Since there is an increasing lag in adaptation to light with age and greater susceptibility to glare, shifts from high to low light values will contribute to confusion and temporary loss of perception. The broad centerline refers to wheelchair users and the dashed line indicates ambulatory users. (From the unpublished study of lighting in nursing home settings by Kieselbach and Hatch, 1975.)

There is no reason why there can't be plantings, mailboxes, lounging chairs, and other means of marking space as well as providing visual and recreational interest (Figure 25).

The corridor should be a kind of siphon, drawing people out of their rooms and into contact with other people, activities, and stimulation in general. Obviously, to accommodate a much larger range of activities, the corridor or space devoted to it must increase. However, spaces devoted to therapy and other specialized functions such as chapels would need to be reallocated so that this concept could be realized. There would be five distinct components of the corridor neighborhood: the promenade area, lounging-activity stations, directional-instructional markers, observation stations, and therapy stations. It would be inherent that these five components are not separate isolated entities but integrated into a whole to provide the stimulation necessary to draw people from their rooms (Figure 25).

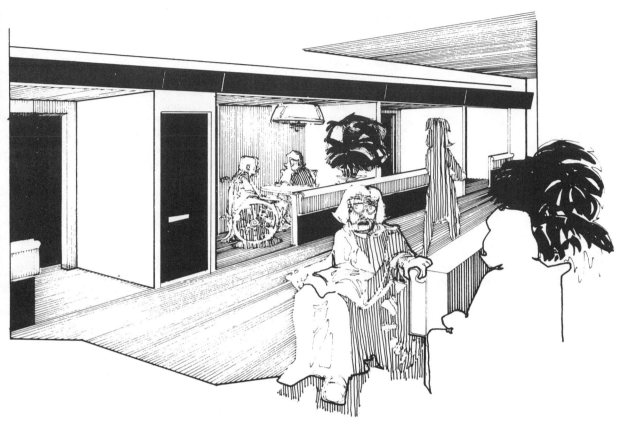

FIGURE 25
Corridor neighborhood. The corridor configuration that uti-
lizes the concept of social space adjoining the room entrance
is really a reflection of the "street, porch, and house" concept of the transition needed to effect interchange. The
passive watcher participating in activity through observation
can be drawn into the activity after absorbing the activity
from a safe distance. There is also tremendous potential for
very attractive corridors that will provide great variety.

Promenade Area

The word "promenade" is chosen deliberately to
convey the sense that walking or in some other way
traversing the corridors should be something done for
pleasure and at leisure. The corridor is usually treated
as a funnel through which the patient-residents are
poured into various activities in other isolated spaces.
To promenade is to enjoy the journey for its own
sake—and much of the therapy conducted in nursing
homes is walking.

For effective stimulation to happen, there must be
appropriate and interesting organizations of the other
elements involved in the corridor design. However,
prior to any further elaborations on the design of the
corridor, there must be careful attention given to
curing some of the oldest problems of corridor design.

One of the most serious problems of the corridor is
the repetition of elements over very long lengths of
hallway. Doorways fall at regular intervals, lighting is
spaced evenly down the center of the ceiling, and
even floor tiles create a regular unbroken pattern,
which seemingly goes into oblivion. Added to the
problem of repetitious elements is the great quantity

of glare off cleaned and shiny surfaces. Where there is exposure to end-of-hall window walls or intermittent windows placed along the corridor, the glare is almost blinding. The elderly eye has serious difficulty adjusting in this environment and perception of where one is with respect to other places may become confused and difficult to judge. The repetition of elements also lends itself to disorienting the patient-resident (Figures 26-30).

The elevator, or vertical transportation mode, in nursing homes is also a contributor to feelings of confusion. Often, the elderly patient–resident will leave one floor on an elevator searching for another, only to be confronted with another floor or several floors all marked in the same way, with the same lighting, wall colors, and floor tile. At the elevator station, an effort could be made to utilize redundant cuing and "supergraphic" symbols to reinforce the little shining light in the elevator that is illuminating the floor number. A simple bell could also be used, which peals for the number of the floor and does so at regular intervals while the elevator doors are open (Figure 31).

The corridor floor surface is an essential part of providing a pleasurable experience. The hardness of tile, its smoothness and glossiness, detract greatly from its use as a suitable floor covering for the nursing home. However, its cleanability, wear resistance, and other factors make it the standard choice among many builders of nursing home space. Carpeting provides excellent feel, attractive surfaces, and almost no glare; but it is more difficult to clean and provides resistance to food carts, which are hard to maneuver and push. Some resistance is also provided to geriatric wheelchairs and wheelchairs, but not in a prohibitive degree. No shag carpeting should ever be used in these types of environments, nor should there be use of deep pile or sculptured pile carpeting. There are commercial-grade carpets and indoor–outdoor carpets that have tight weaves and low pile. These are the more appropriate choices if carpets are chosen for corridors.

The backing of the carpet is as important as the carpet itself. Some of the backing materials give off noxious fumes when they burn and also black smoke. The manufacturers of the products should be con-

tacted about product specifications to make an appropriate choice.

Because of the great variety of carpets and the number of variations that can be made throughout a facility and the tremendous glare reduction, greater use of carpets should be made. The feel of a carpet and its noise reduction factor also make it very important in capturing a sense of pleasure in walking or moving through the corridor neighborhood. The cleaning problems seem less prohibitive as time passes. Industrial cleaning techniques could solve this problem. Consider the problem of cleaning an artificial turf football field as an example.

Lighting of the corridor should be carefully controlled from both the standpoint of quantity of light and glare reduction. In double-loaded corridors, natural light penetrates only at the end of the corridor and at any interval between rooms leading off the corridor. The corridor is then dimly lit, in most instances, using artificial light, and the result is a dark tunnel with very bright glaring ends or intermittent hot spots.

It is probably better to screen out natural lighting from the corridor because of its interference with the necessity to see the surroundings and identify various markers. The variation using natural unbaffled or unfiltered daylight is so great as to be a hindrance to sight in the dimmer corridor.

There should be more effective use of indirect peripheral lighting in corridors. Lights placed down the center of the corridor may have the virtue of accessibility for maintenance, but they do not effectively provide a sense of the walls as boundaries nor do they highlight identification areas on walls. There has been some use of indirect lighting used behind handrails. This sets off the handrail from the wall and clearly marks it for use by those who need to use it. This use of lighting also marks the juncture of the floor and wall and provides a sense of the total width of the hallway (Figure 32). Just as in the patient–resident room, balanced lighting or careful judicious choices of fluorescent lighting must be made to avoid giving a blue-green cast to the overall corridor and to maximize flattering the flesh tones of those using the corridors. As stated in the chapter on the physiological aspects

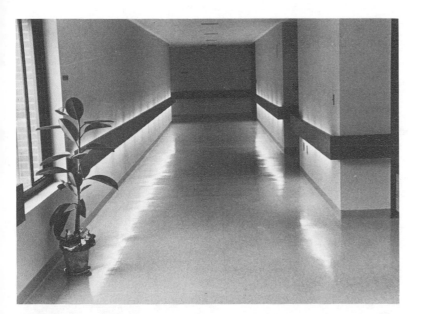

FIGURE 26
Corridor studies. Glare, sameness, lack of orientating graphics, and little liveliness often characterize the typical institutional corridor. However, Figures 26 and 27 show an innovative use of the handrail as a barrier to prevent abrasion from carts and indirect illumination from lighting recessed in the handrail, beyond contact. The handrails are also mounted at 26 inches from the floor to the top edge, which permits greater use by non-ambulatory patient-residents, over 70 percent of the resident population in this institution. (Photo: John Kelsey and Robert Steinbugler.)

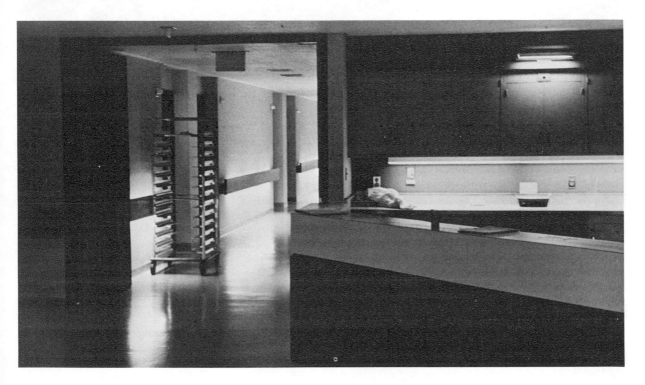

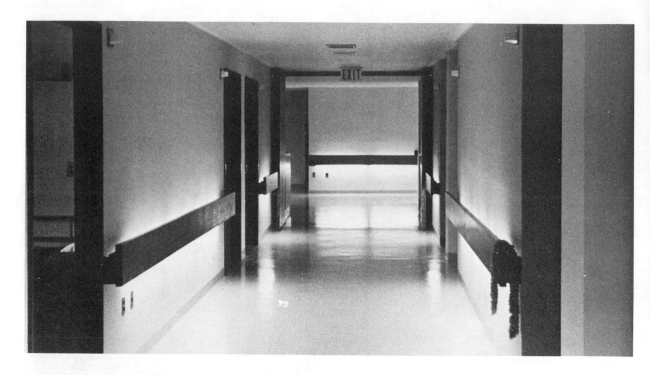

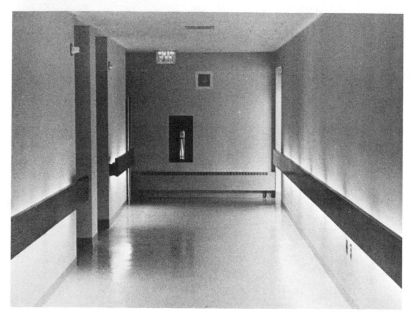

FIGURE 27
Corridor studies. There must be a more concerted effort to place identifying "place" markers in corridors. Lack of proper identifying graphics often leads to confusion for many lucid, but sensorily infirm, patient–residents. (Photo: John Kelsey and Robert Steinbugler.)

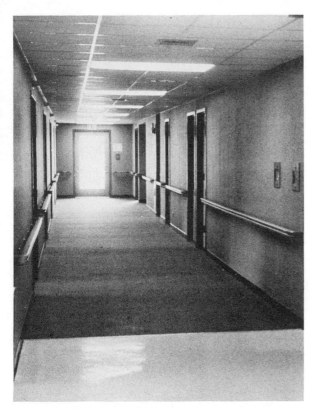

FIGURE 28
Corridor study. There can be a significant reduction of glare when carpeting is installed in corridors. (Photo: John Kelsey and Robert Steinbugler.)

of aging, the blue-green range of colors are the most difficult to perceive for the aging eye. A total cast of blue-green in the corridor might add further confusion for the users of this space.

All corridors in nursing homes are required to provide a handrail mounted to the wall to support those who need to grasp a rigid support while they walk. However, there is much confusion over just what the most appropriate handrail should be like and at what height it should be mounted. Heights from the floor vary in nursing homes from 26 to 39 inches. Cross sections vary from circular with a diameter of ¾ inch to rectilinear shapes of varying dimensions. The largest number of handrails are circular cross sections of about 2 inches in diameter mounted about 32 inches from the floor. This follows the recommendation of the President's Committee on Employment of the Handicapped, Recommendations of the Subcommittee on Barrier Free Design (ANSI Standard 117.1) (1971) (Figure 32) and also Goldsmith's (1967, pages 70-71) recommendations.

Observations of activity in corridors have given rise to the premise that a minority of ambulatory patient-residents actually use the handrail for assistance while walking. The predominant use of the handrail in nursing homes is by the nonambulatory patient-residents who pull themselves down the corridor using the handrail as an ambulatory assist. This means that a large number of handrails are mounted too high for the people who actually use them.

A problem associated with the use of the handrails in this manner is the high rate of scuffing and marking of the wall surfaces because of the wheelchairs turning inward with each pull along the rail. There should be a barrier at the low wheel level to prevent the wheelchair from turning inward far enough to hit the wall.

To optimize the design of handrails in corridors, it is possible that a double handrail should be worked out with a barrier or kickplate at the base of the wall to prevent scuffing. One handrail should be at 32 inches and the other at approximately 26 inches to allow for use by both the ambulatory and nonambulatory. Since this scheme becomes more complex, it is likely that an integrated lighting system with the handrail could be worked out which would mark the width of the corridor and show the scuff plate at the wall base to prevent tripping (Figure 32).

Visual and Textural Markers

There are two aspects to the use of visual and textural elements in the corridor: identification of place and environmental enrichment. There are both overt and subtle ways to communicate the location of various parts of a building. Signs with arrows are the more typical method employed to direct people. However, the placement of a plant or picture, the change of light on the surface of a wall, even noises and smells let people know where they are in relation

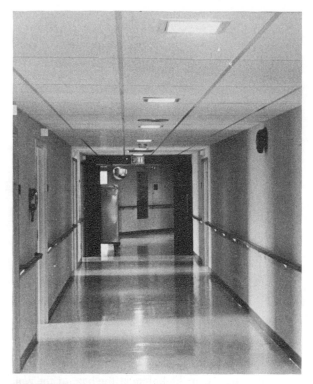

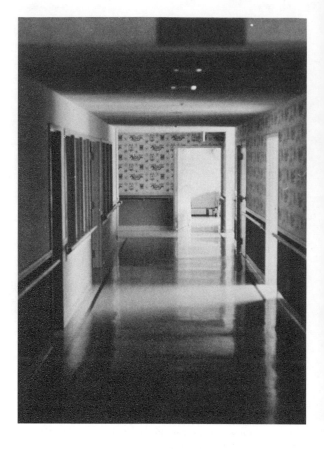

FIGURE 29
Corridor studies. Glare can be a problem regardless of the light level. While photographs can be deceptive, the light levels are noticeably different in the two corridors shown, yet the reflectance from the floor surfaces is still a factor in both corridors. (Photo: John Kelsey and Robert Steinbugler.)

to other places or where they want to be. Along with the use of various devices to mark space, these same devices also enrich space and give it attractiveness. It is interesting to see how devoid of visual and textural richness most modern nursing homes are and especially how monotonous the corridors (Figure 29).

Insufficient use of textures is the state of things in most nursing homes. While textures have great unexplored value as elements used to identify space, most designers and builders rely on visual messages alone to convey location. One texture predominates in the corridors of most nursing homes—high-gloss smooth surfaces to infinity. There should be plantings, sculp-

tures, and appropriate drapery materials to curb the monotonous effect of lack of texture.

In terms of the use of textures to identify space, marking the handrail with either a change of surface or dips and raises in the surface could indicate location to the partially sighted and the blind. A system of textural codes, like braille, could be designed to convey position and location. Subtle changes could be made to floor surfaces or to corners of walls, which could bend around from one corridor to the next to reinforce these changes in the environment.

Visual markers have received some attention with the use of signs and graphics to mark corridor and

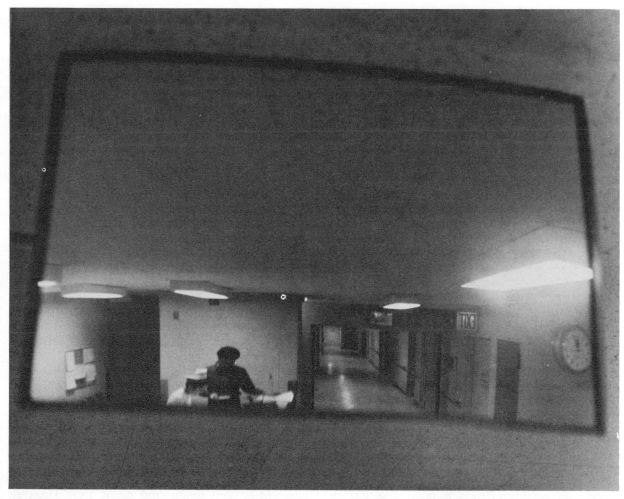

FIGURE 30

Corridor study. One of the most direct solutions to the problem of visual access for both patient-residents and staff is the provision of mirrors at critical intersections and juxtaposed from nursing stations. (Photo: David O. Watkins.)

room locations. Color coding of doorsills has also been attempted with varying degrees of success. One problem with color coding is that it must be bold enough and striking enough to convey differences from any other element in the immediate surroundings. There is also nothing wrong with telling the occupants of a corridor neighborhood about the various methods used to identify their space. It may be asking too much of the system that it be self-explanatory (Figure 33).

Color coding and supergraphics are not the only means of conveying a message visually; pictures could be mounted to the doors of patient-residents to show who lives within. The pictures need not be of the patient-residents, but should be carefully screened so that confusion doesn't reign.

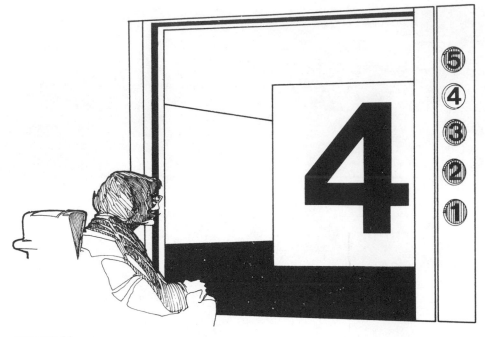

FIGURE 31
View from the elevator. When the doors open, the floor should be clearly and boldly marked. A great many possibilities exist for the graphic treatment of corridors and floor levels.

Visual markers should also be used to denote areas within the environment of the corridor to give them distinctive character. A change in the direction of a hallway, the halfway point in the corridor itself, and other areas may be repeated on floor after floor of a physical environment. Visual markers such as color changes or bright color areas, paintings, plantings, or other devices could be used to provide a sense of which of the various floors any given floor might be. This could be helpful to the patient–resident who needs signposts as reminders as well as constant memory jogs—or redundant cues.

Lounging-Activity Stations

As stated in the chapter on planning, there is no denying that lounging and other recreational activities take place in the corridor. This must be viewed as an encumbrance in the traditional corridor because there is no provision made for anything except mobility and transport. However, provision should be made for activities in the corridor as a recognition of the complex set of functions that are found there and cannot be wished or regulated out of existence. There should be an 8-foot free, unencumbered space for mobility and transport adjoining the isolated spaces, such as patient–resident rooms, and dining areas. However, outside of this space, the periphery should not be the constant repetition of blank walls. There should be articulations of the surfaces adjoining the corridor space so that small areas can be set aside for arrangements of tables and chairs or chairs alone. Some areas might have plantings; others might be large enough to accommodate one or two patient-residents for eating their meals.

The precise arrangement of this type of space vis-a-vis the entrance to patient-residents' rooms and other isolated spaces could vary greatly. A plan used with some frequency is to build in a central service core of rooms with corridors on two sides and the patient-

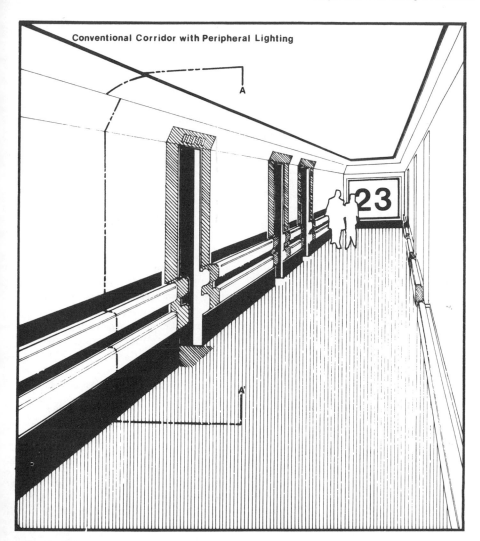

Conventional Corridor with Peripheral Lighting

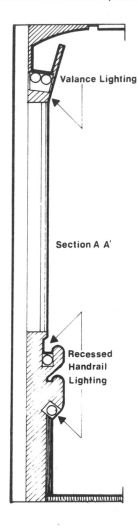

Valance Lighting

Section A A'

Recessed
Handrail
Lighting

FIGURE 32

Conventional corridor. Many possibilities exist for the treatment of the conventional corridor beyond the characteristics usually associated with their institutional quality. One of the most significant changes should come in the treatment of lighting. Greater use of indirect lighting should be planned along with careful selection of light quality. Color coding of corridors to promote ease of identification (including corridor numbering) and double handrails for wheelchair users are advisable steps toward effective change.

residents' rooms to the outside of the corridors. The central core of this type of plan could also be changed to incorporate these lounging-activity stations. Another possibility is to have the entrance area of each patient–resident room become the lounging-activity station. This could be considered a kind of "front porch" concept, with the corridor promenade area becoming an avenue (Figure 25).

The possibilities of spatial arrangements and arrangements of furnishings extend to the concept of a large

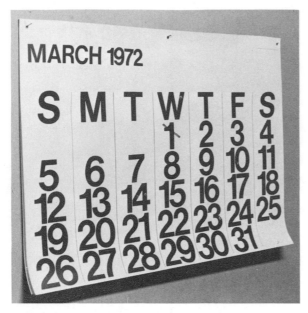

FIGURE 33
Corridor study. A large-print calendar is functioning as a signpost in thus nursing home corridor. (Photo: David O. Watkins.)

central court bordered by a corridor or free unimpeded space. The central court, in essence a kind of park, would embrace all the functions of the facility outside of the patient–resident room. This type of plan is often referred to as the "sociopetal" plan; the patient–resident is provided every amenity within one unit of the facility without the use of isolated spaces in other sections of the physical environment. This means that the patient–resident sees or is near activity throughout the day, and is drawn into that activity either to participate actively or passively.

To return to the concept of the lounging–activity station, the point is not to replace the lounge or the special therapy room where personal and private attention can be given to one person, but to recognize that much of the passive activity and indeed much of the therapy given in a facility happens right outside the patient–residents' doors. The accommodation of these functions and activities provides interesting possibilities for new and original configurations of

space and possibilities for treating these spaces (see Figures 34–37).

Observation Stations

The nursing station in the traditional nursing home is a source of stimulation for many of the patient–residents who gravitate to the location of the station to watch the activity taking place there on a continuing basis. Likewise, one of the more important aspects of the nursing station in the facility is that it is the place from which activity in the halls can be watched. Yet, a great number of the nursing stations built into the corridors of nursing homes are either recessed from the hallway or in some other way placed so that observation of activity is difficult or impossible from the station itself. It should be possible for the nurse on duty at the nursing station to monitor the activity going on in the hallway space of which the nursing station is a part. It is also important that nursing stations be located or planned for a facility in such number and position so that all corridors can be monitored by the nurse on duty without the nurse having to leave the station (Figures 38 and 39).

Thus the term "nursing station" is not really appropriate to the function. "Observation station" would signify a recognition of the most important function the nursing station fulfills.

Therapy Stations

Very frequently, the least used space within a facility is the physical therapy room. While examining rooms are frequently used for treating patient–residents, the physical therapy room is not the active beehive of rehabilitation that regulations seem to specify or indicate. One problem associated with the use of special rooms and specialized retraining devices is that their function is actually a duplication of the function that the rest of the facility provides on a constant and continuing basis. It is the lower extremities of the body that need rebuilding or retraining in a great number of cases, or exercise in relation to the use of the large motor muscles that is required. Most of the space in the nursing home can be so designed to accommodate the needs of those requiring physiotherapy training or assistance. Steps can be located in

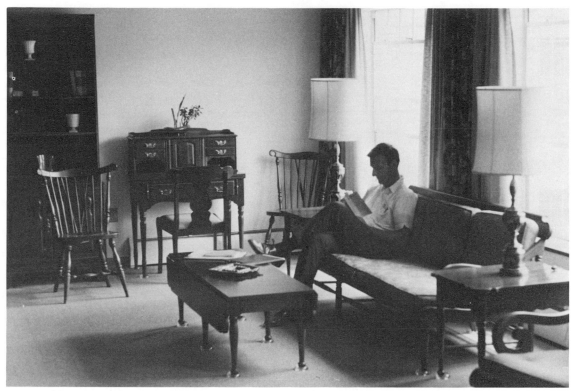

FIGURE 34

Lounge study. This nursing home lounge functions mainly as a visitors' lobby. It is not accessible to patient–residents, but gives the impression of a homelike setting. The other lounges in this particular institution are not carpeted, nor do they contain as many carefully chosen and placed furnishings. (Photo: John Kelsey and Robert Steinbugler.)

part of the corridor and made accessible to only those requiring their use. The design of this specialized instrument should be modified to reduce its clinical appearance. It could become a bridge crossing an arrangement of plantings surrounding a small pool—anything that might provide a visual, tactile, olfactory, or general sensory reward for partaking of the effort and journey to accomplish essentially a rehabilitation-orientated exercise (Figure 25).

The Philadelphia Geriatric Center, using a modified sociopetal plan for a new nursing home unit, incorporates a gazebo in a large, open lounge–activity center. Entering and egressing the gazebo is a climbing maneuver with a sensory reward because of the at-

tractiveness of the device. The gazebo is accessible to all patient-residents, but is obviously intended as a device to be used for supervised rehabilitation exercises.

Corridors are often used as rehabilitation areas because there is considerable effort needed to get patient-residents into wheelchairs, transported to special rooms, and transferred out of the chairs for the exercise. This also spawns considerable anticipation or anxiety on the part of the patient-resident, which is not conducive to a good rehabilitative session. Therefore, the corridor, with its handrail in place, is often the site of many rehabilitation sessions.

Once again, creating therapy stations in the corridor

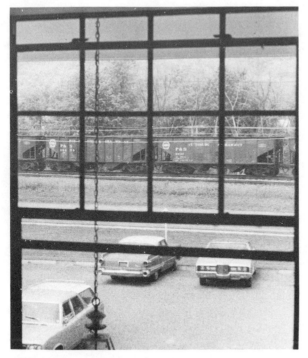

FIGURE 35
Lounge study. In the same facility as that shown in Figure 34 is a second-floor lounge endowed with visual riches from the window. The movement of the trains and the activity in the parking lot are extremely attractive stimuli for passive watching. (Photo: John Kelsey and Robert Steinbugler.)

complex is really a recognition of the activities already taking place in a good many nursing homes simply because it is the easiest, least traumatic, and most natural use of the facility. There is also likely to be greater acceptance of the rehabilitation program if patient–residents can see it functioning around them, and it is a natural and rewarding experience.

Occupational therapy is essentially designed to exercise the small motor muscles in the arms and retrain after trauma or paralysis to improve or rebuild the use of the hand for manipulative skills. However, there is another aspect of the typical occupational therapy program in nursing homes: it is an activity with an object orientation, a beginning and an end,

and the special reward of having created something tangible. It is not accidental that the largest majority of "activity" programs seem to be offshoots of occupational therapy programs or developments from the specific tasks of occupational therapy. Basket weaving, fabric weaving on looms, ceramic casting, and the like, are all used as both occupational therapy as well as general activity practices. General activity should *not* be limited to occupational therapy programs as a resource, but there is values in the translation of these activities into more general participation (Figure 40).

The point is that these activities are very attractive to watch as well as participate in. They are drawing cards, which can stimulate the reluctant patient–resident to participate in activities, at least passively, if these activities can be seen and are readily accessible.

The actual separation, either visually or environmentally, of the general-use lounge–activity stations and the occupational therapy stations may not be distinguishable, nor need it be. The definition of difference between these two functions need not be environmental but be a function of the utilization of staff and specific assistance, help, or instruction given to specific patient–residents.

Another important therapy function being conducted in a great many nursing homes is called reality training or reality therapy. It consists generally of training sessions with specially trained staff in which patient–residents with chronic brain syndrome are encouraged to recognize where they are, who they are, what they are doing, what day it is, and so on. The essence of this continuing therapy is to promote mental involvement and to fight off progressive mental deterioration to whatever degree possible for the individual patient–resident. Some patient–residents respond remarkably to this constant jogging of the mental processes, while others do not respond at all (Figure 41).

The predictability and actual effects of reality therapy are not clear and there is argument about its validity. However, for patient–residents who are afflicted with chronic brain syndrome (catchall for a variety of symptoms and an even greater variety of

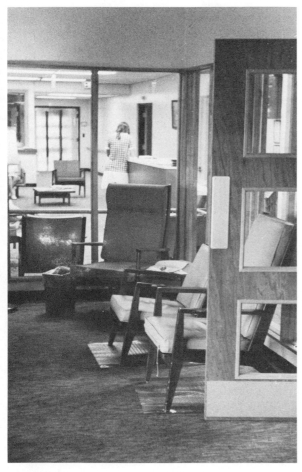

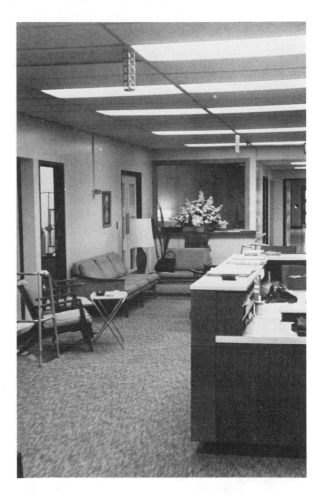

FIGURE 36

Lobby–lounge study. A relatively small facility consolidated several functional interior components and amenities in one central lobby–lounge. Adjacent to this space is another lounge with a glass wall permitting visual access to the lobby–lounge. Both areas are highly utilized because they have so much potential for passive watching (see Figure 37). Notice the plastic sheets under the geriatric chairs to protect the carpeting against incontinence. (Photo: John Kelsey and Robert Steinbugler.)

psychological impairments), there are few activities in which they can participate, and this daily constancy of sessions is helpful as something to be anticipated and as positive involvement. Otherwise, there is nothing available in nursing homes to involve these people.

Reality training sessions are reinforced through environmental stimuli placed throughout the facility. Signs, calendars, and other devices are used to relate the patient–residents to time, place, and activity. At present, the physical devices that accompany reality therapy are not planned into the design from the

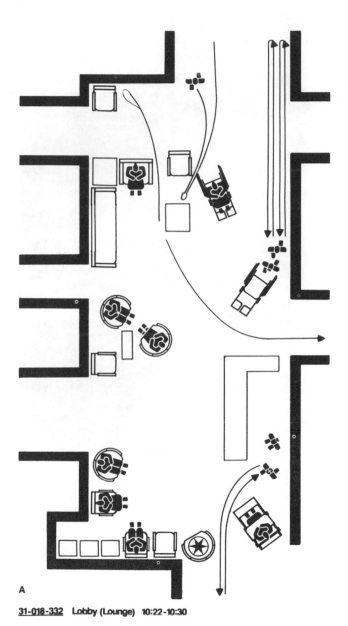

A

<u>31-018-332</u>   Lobby (Lounge)   10:22-10:30

FIGURE 37

A. Lobby-lounge with limited activity; B. Lobby-lounge with high activity. The configuration of space and various functional components in space act as a siphon, drawing residents into the lobby-lounge to watch and perhaps to par-

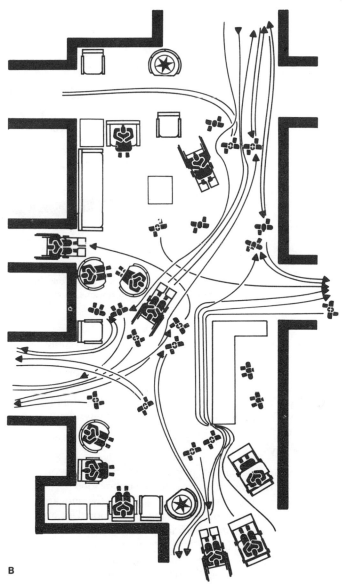

B

<u>31-018-332</u> Lobby (Lounge) 10:30-10:50; <u>31-019-332</u> 10:33-10:50

ticipate. However, owing to the multiplicity of directions from which activity can generate, there is a general confusion and frequent blockage of passage.

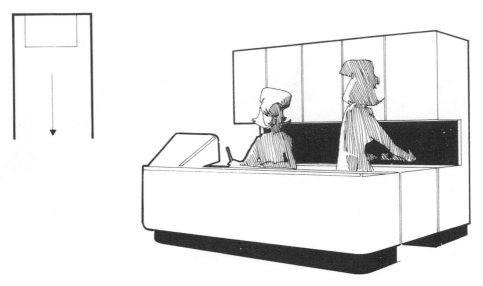

FIGURE 38
Nursing station. Nursing stations must provide visual access down the corridor for the nursing staff to monitor activity. In new design development, corridors should be shorter with the terminal ends housing the nursing stations. In existing buildings, there should be greater use of mirrors carefully located for monitoring.

beginning. However, this could be done and also could serve as part of the overall programing of the visual markers that are placed throughout the corridor system. Large-print calendars and other signs could be used by anyone, but could be serving the double purpose of therapy for some of the patient-residents.

Lounge Bays

One essential changes that it is necessary to incorporate if the idea of a corridor neighborhood is to take shape in the nursing home facility is the annexation of space usually delegated to the traditional isolated lounge. Reasons for this change have been discussed at an earlier stage in the text. However, it suffices to say that the idea of a corridor neighborhood would not succeed if lounges remain the way they are (Figure 42).

Lounges do not presently meet their intended purpose, that is, the promotion of socialization among patient-residents and the providing of a place of re-

treat or relaxation. For a large number of patient-residents, present lounges are inaccessible, impeded within by furniture unsuitable for use by most of the patient-residents, and so far from bathroom facilities as to be unsatisfactory for use by those who are anxious about their ability to control excretory functions.

Therefore, as part of the concept of the corridor neighborhood, there should be intermittent breaks in the space of the promenade area where larger groups of people can gather yet still have visual access and immediate participation in the activity outside of these spaces. These spaces would be appropriately known as "bays," because they are shelter away from the current of activity, the flow of traffic in the corridor itself.

In these bays, there should be minimum of fixed furnishings—furnishings that remain in the space to accommodate users. The majority of the users are going to be in wheelchairs or geriatric wheelchairs, and excessive amounts of side chairs or other seating

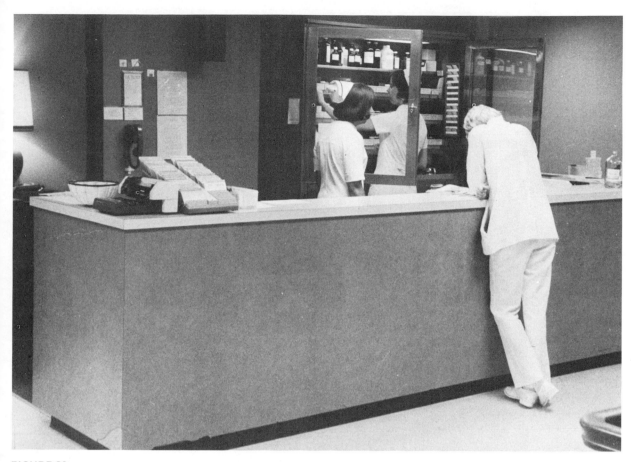

FIGURE 39

Nursing station. While this station is removed from an area providing sufficient room for watching behavior, it is still frequented by a high number of patient–residents. Notice the scuffing damage to the lower-left edge of the front panel. (Photo: John Kelsey and Robert Steinbugler.)

meant for the ambulatory will impede the free use of this space. Likewise, all tables should be of the 30-inch variety with minimal aprons to facilitate use by the nonambulatory. If the bay happens to be situated with an exterior window wall, the tables should be moved to a position near the windows so that conversational groupings can move near a focus of interest on the outside, yet still have the advantages the table provides both for activities that require a surface and for the visual protection mentioned earlier.

The lounge bay should have some focus of interest in the space as well as being a protected alcove away from activity. Television watching, additional plantings, aquaria, song birds, and other possibilities arise because of the protection afforded in this area.

There should be access to a bathroom very near the lounge bay. In the observations of Koncelik et al. (1972), very few facilities had bathrooms near the lounge, and this was a fairly consistent complaint of the patient-residents interviewed.

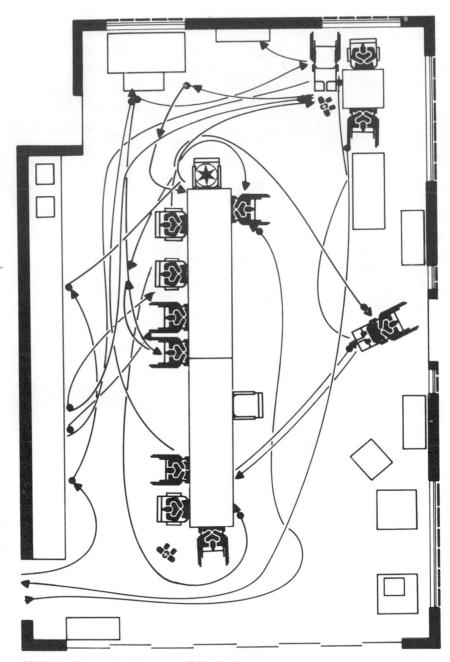

23-OOI-III **Recreational Therapy** IO:IO-IO:45

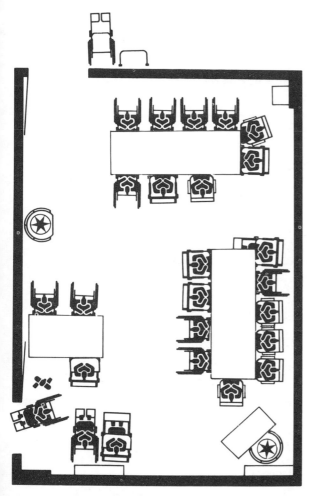

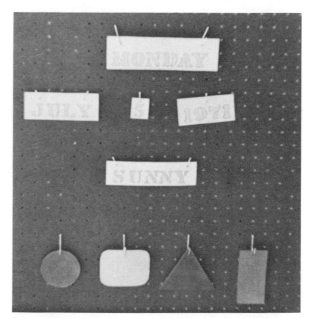

FIGURE 41
Reality training instruction board. The effectiveness and the quality of reality therapy fluctuates widely among the nursing homes that employ it, but there is evidence of success. However, the tools used in many instances are primitive; they need careful, considerate design attention. There should be a better system of graphic symbols, which are more visible and distinguishable from one another. (Photo: John Kelsey and Robert Steinbugler.)

FIGURE 40 (*left and above*)
Recreational therapy–activity therapy. Some forms of activity that require active participation are best provided within a designated space, but not all activity should be so offered. The "ganged" activities usually mean that there is little possibility for variation during the session. Everyone is constrained by the number of people in a group activity.

Figures 43–53 illustrate types of lounges and many of the pitfalls to be avoided in their design.

DINING ROOMS

It is important to recognize that not all the consumption of food at meals is going to take place in the dining room. In some facilities as few as 50 percent of the residents, and sometimes fewer, use the dining rooms for their meals. There are a variety of reasons for this. The bedridden cannot get to the dining room; many of the less able or chronic brain syndrome patient-residents eat in their rooms or are fed either in their rooms or in the corridors just outside their rooms. However, for a sizable number of patient-residents, especially for the ambulatory or others who are inclined to socialize at mealtime and look forward to the meal as an event, the dining room is an important place.

The dining space should be more isolated than the lounge bay because the focus of attention is the meal itself and the companionship of the people who are partaking of the meal with each other. Here again,

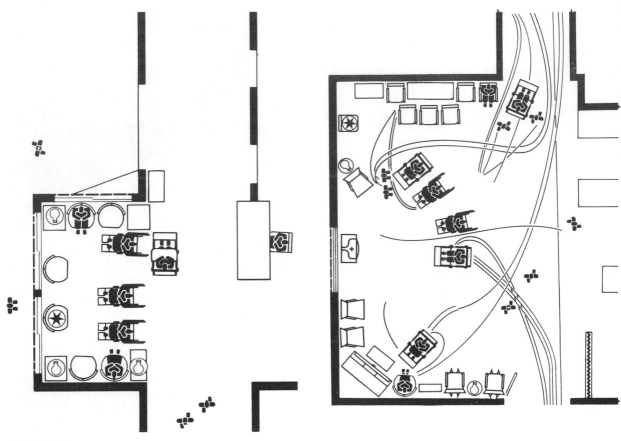

FIGURE 42

Lounge bays. One of the greatest assets of the lounge with an open end off the corridor is that it can act as a way station and buffer activity zone. However, as can be seen, lounge bays should not be impeded by placing too much unusable furniture in these spaces.

however, the dining spaces usually found in the traditional nursing home are too large, noisy, and inconvenient for traffic flow. Dining rooms should be smaller, perhaps one dining room per wing seating no more than 15 to 20 people at one sitting (Figure 54).

A good deal of attention should be paid to the decor of the dining room, not only from the standpoint of esthetics but also because of the need to reduce sound or abate background noise. Although carpeting would not be recommended in these spaces because of food spillage, fabric wall hangings, acoustic panels in the ceiling, and other devices should be explored so that the problem of noise can be reduced.

In lieu of investigations with tables of various sizes in combination to form dining spaces, the four-position table seems the most suitable for the purposes of grouping, entrance and egress from the table position, and from the room space. If a six-position table is used in dining rooms, there will be at least one back-to-back arrangement that cannot be avoided, promulgating conflicts in extracting the occupants of these two spaces, especially if either or both hap-

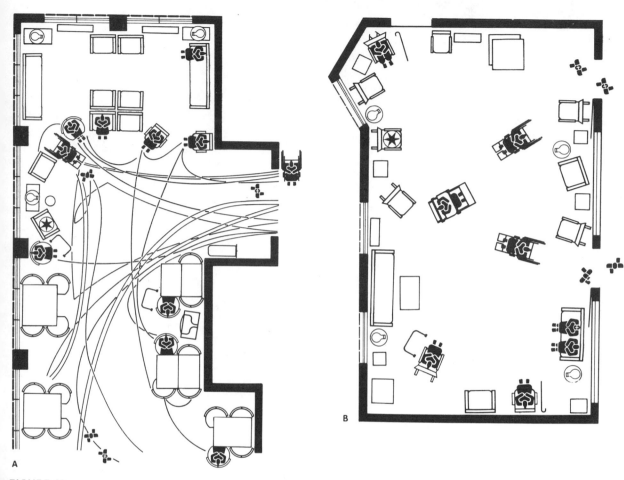

FIGURE 43

A. Lounge with inherent traffic pattern. B. Isolated–enclosed lounge. Both maps represent lounges that are independent and enclosed spaces. The first incorporates a traffic pattern and the second does not. In the first, the room occupants carefully place themselves so that they can passively observe the action along the traffic pattern out to the elevators. In the second, there is too little room for movement and congregation of nonambulatory room occupants. Notice again the disuse of furnishings meant for the ambulatory, although not as dramatic as later maps portray.

pen to be in wheelchairs or in geriatric chairs (Figures 54 and 55).

The shape of the table is a matter of preferences rather than subject to any clear indication that square is better than round, or vice versa. Round tables can be approached from any angle without the impedence of a sharp corner. Some researchers argue that the square table allows the occupant to mark off definite territory (Sommer, 1969). Yet the round table allows for a certain amount of flexibility; another table occupant can join a group with adjustments to the seating positions for every occupant—equalization of spaces occupied—instead of just two persons being crowded at one end of the table.

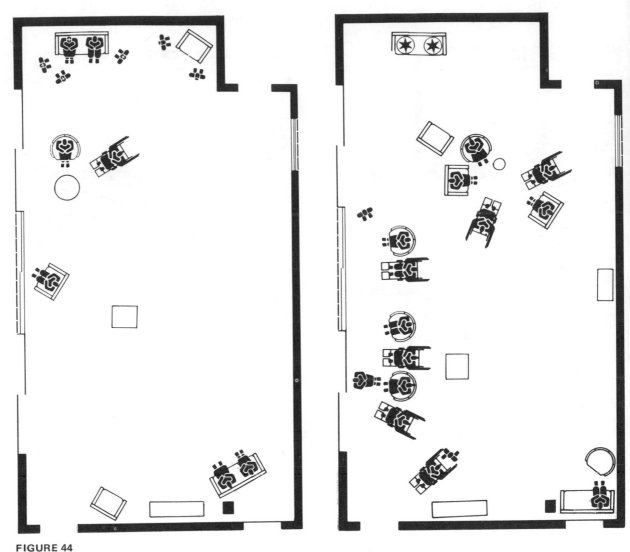

FIGURE 44

Flexible multifunctional lounge. With sufficient space for movement and few furnishings to clog the space, there is greater opportunity to form clusters, as shown in the right map, independent of the constraints imposed by improper furniture.

All dining chairs that are free standing and not a device fixed to the table should have arms. These arms both support and constrain. The arms should penetrate beneath the surface of the table or the support apron between the legs (see Figure 56). It is surprising to see how many chairs and table combina-

tions, supposedly matched sets, do not meet this recommendation. Designers and buyers of equipment for facilities should be very aware that this problem exists with a good share of institutional furnishings on the market. Another problem is that many tables are too low to accommodate wheelchairs or geriatric

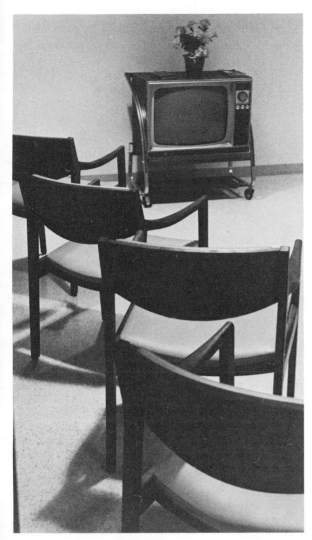

FIGURE 45
Television lounge. (Photo: John Kelsey and Robert Steinbugler.)

FIGURE 46
Unifunctional space. Space devoted to one function or activity
is not a sound planning or designing practice. Observations
on use of television lounges indicate that their use is minimal.
Smaller more intimate lounges have desirable characteristics,
but they should remain multifunctional.

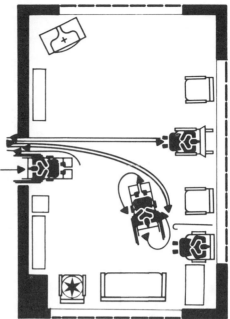

21-OO6-221 Corridor Lounge 10:25-10:55

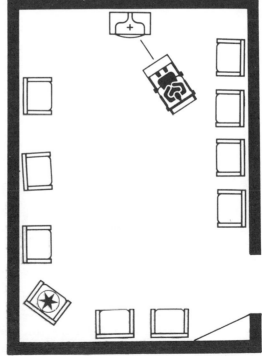

71-094-211 Corridor Television Lounge 3:15-3:30

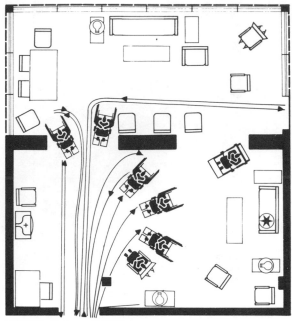

21-002-131 Corridor Lounge 10:36-11:25

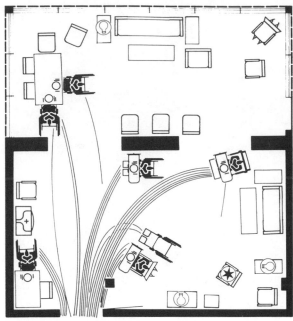

21-016-121 Corridor Lounge 12:30-1:15

FIGURE 47 (*left, above, and right*)

Corridor lounge with solarium. A corridor lounge is a lounge space that is adjacent to or at the end of a corridor. A single lounge is represented over time in these mapping studies. Several problems are evident. First, access into the lounge is across the television viewing area, which results in a serious congestion of the space. Second, the brightness of the solarium and the preponderance of furniture meant for the ambulatory, except when there is feeding. It is rather obvious that some adjustments to the furnishings arrangement could help to free up the access and possibly increase the utilization of the solarium space.

wheelchairs. It would be optimum if a table and chair combination could be designed that would suit the wheelchairs and geriatric chairs as well.

BATHROOMS

There is a need for a controlled environment where assisted bathing, nursing, examination, and treatment can take place. This type of bathroom is a specialized environment, not to be treated as a community bathroom. The special nature of this place requires spe-

cialized equipment. Unfortunately, the specialized equipment currently available for this type of bathing area is outdated and needs serious study and redevelopment. The hoyer lift, for example, is a device used to lift the disabled from the bed or from a chair and transport them to the bathroom where they can be bathed. This piece of equipment, the method of operation, and other facets of its use make it a very poor and dangerous piece of equipment for nursing home use. The bathtub should not be a standard model basically intended for residential use, but higher

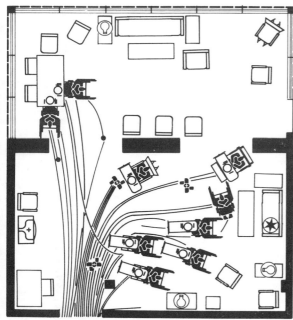

21-017-221 Corridor Lounge 12:30-1:15

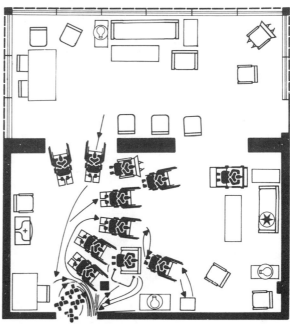

21-004-231 Corridor Lounge 10:00-10:30

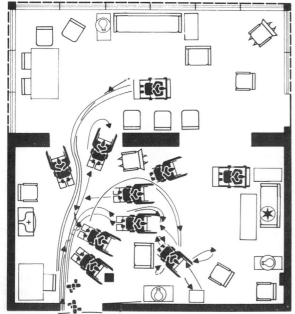

21-004-231 Corridor Lounge 10:30-11:00

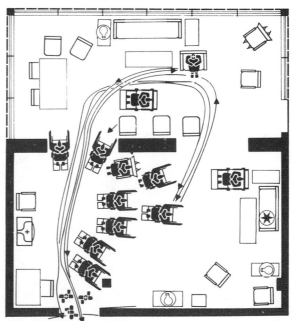

21-004-231 Corridor Lounge 11:00-11:20

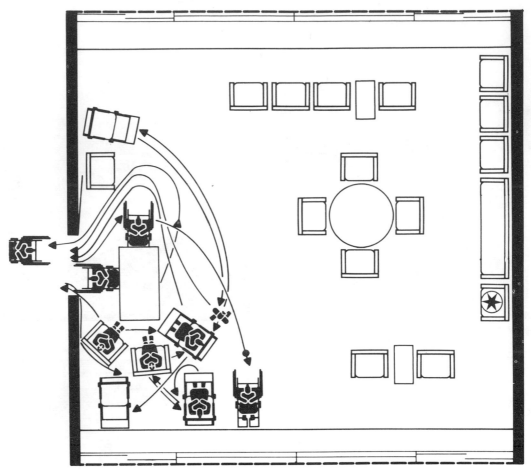

71-080-251 Corridor Lounge 12:30-1:30

FIGURE 48

Corridor lounge with unworkable furniture. One nursing home provided an extraordinary opportunity for study because it had several large lounge spaces all furnished and maintained in precisely the same manner. In this first study of one of these spaces, the conflict between the use of the lounge and the furniture provided to enable utilization is readily seen.

off the floor and, if at all possible, equipped with a seated configuration so that the legs need not be completely extended for some of the patient-residents. Figures 57 and 58 show some problems encountered in bathroom design.

Privacy is extremely important and care should be taken to screen off effectively one bathing–treatment area from another. The same principle holds for the toilets installed in these areas as well.

The floor surface is another extremely important

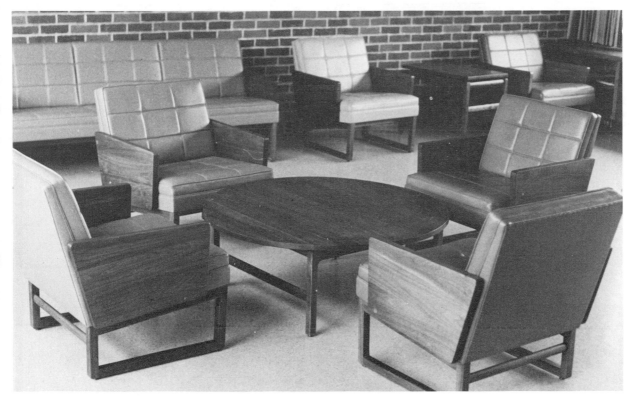

FIGURE 49

Furnishings in a solarium. Though straightforward in design, these chairs and other furnishings are inappropriate for use by an aging infirm population. There is little use of the furnishings as seen in Figures 46–48. (Photo: John Kelsey and Robert Steinbugler.)

area of concern because water spillage is a problem in this area and slipping can be a serious problem. Another factor is the treatment of the entrance doorway with regard to water spillage and buildup. A high sill will impede a lift mechanism upon entrance, yet water spillage into the corridor must be restrained, especially when corridors are carpeted. It is recommended that floor surfaces in these specialized bathrooms be contoured very gradually with a rise at the entrance and low sill (if any need be used at all) to prevent the seepage of water into the hallway.

Bathrooms are also necessary near the public spaces

in the nursing home. It is recommended that a bath be placed next to lounges and dining rooms so that those needing these facilities have immediate access. A lavatory and toilet with sufficient space for a wheelchair to be moved for transfer is a requirement. The same characteristics regarding the grab rails apply here as in the bath in the patient–resident room.

It is possible that use of public spaces is restricted and constrained by the lack of bathroom facilities near them. Patient–residents may feel uneasy using a lounge or dining room when they are so far removed

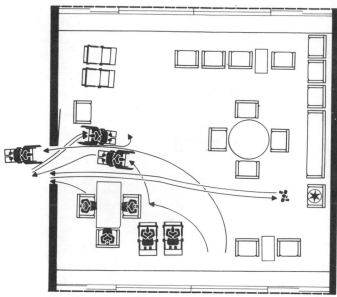

71-081-251 Corridor Lounge 2:07-2:37

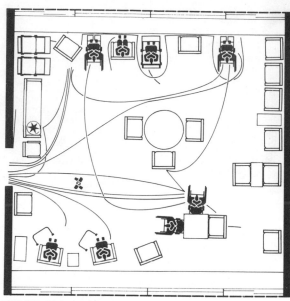

71-090-141 Corridor Lounge 10:45-11:15

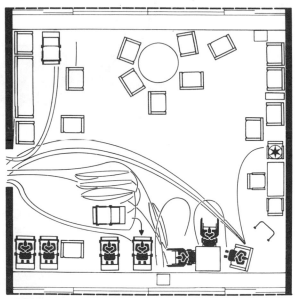

71-086-121 Corridor Lounge 10:30-11:00

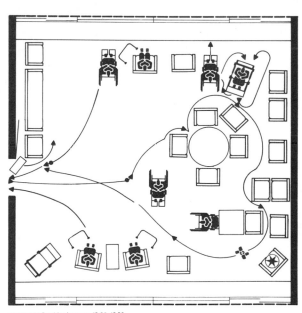

71-092-241 Corridor Lounge 10:00-10:30

FIGURE 50 (*above and right*)

Corridor lounges with the same furniture and arrangement of furnishings. While there is occasional use of some of the furnishings meant for the ambulatory, the furniture is generally unused and the arrangement is unsatisfactory for inter-action or activities. First, owing to the nonambulatory status of the majority of patient--residents, room occupants are placed by others; they rarely choose their own locations. Second, these locations are frequently near the doorway to

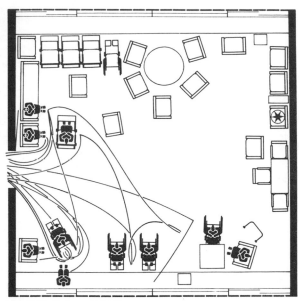

71-087-121 Corridor Lounge 2:30-3:00

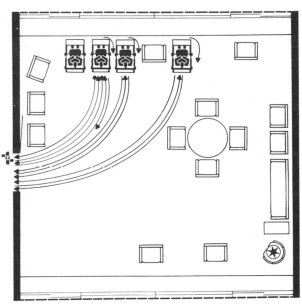

71-082-141 Corridor Lounge 2:45-3:10

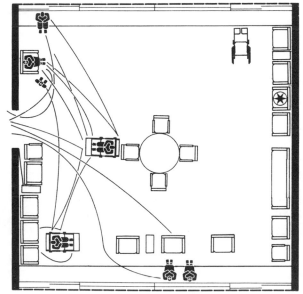

72-088-721 Corridor Lounge 11:50-12:22+

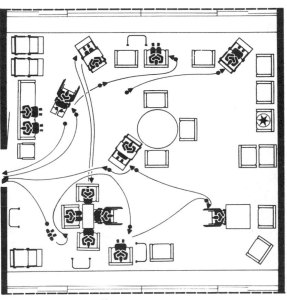

71-093-241 Corridor Lounge 2:15-2:55

permit ease of observation by the staff. Third, owing to the disuse of the spaces, they are taking on the function of storerooms for unused wheelchairs and geriatric wheelchairs.

The low coffee table is of interest because no nonambulatory person can reach down to its surface; it is largely disfunctional.

103

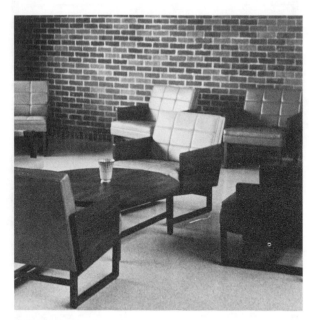

FIGURE 51
An expensive way to use lounge furnishings. (Photo: John Kelsey and Robert Steinbugler.)

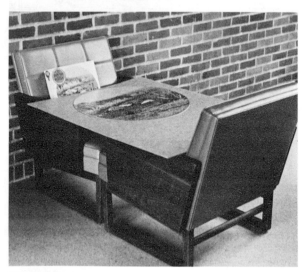

FIGURE 52
An expensive way to use lounge chairs. (Photo: John Kelsey and Robert Steinbugler.)

from a bathroom. As stated previously, it could also be the reason why a large number of patient–residents remain close to their rooms most of the time.

ENTRANCE AREAS

The access passageway to the outside is an important area in nursing homes and other facilities for the aging from the standpoint of its use by the occupants. This area includes the external part of the building from the drive, curb, walkway, and steps to the door, and inside to the reception area, lounge bay, and instruction or direction area. It is surprising to see how many nursing homes fail to consider shrouding the entrance way to protect their clients from the elements upon egress from a car or ambulance. Considering that many of the patient-residents entering a nursing home for the first time are in wheelchairs, it is disturbing to realize that these people are exposed to the elements in the large majority of entrance ways until they reach the door. The expense added to the architecture of a building to shroud the entrance way up to the point of the curb cannot be prohibitive and is an important design consideration.

There should be no steps leading up to the entrance or doorway. Once again, however, even contemporary nursing homes are still employing the use of steps at the entrance to the facility. This should be considered an architectural barrier of the first order for this kind of construction—steps should be eliminated. There should also be support rails out to the point of the curb for support while walking. Indeed, the external environmental conditions are more dangerous at times than the interior environment. There is phenomenal glare; walkways are usually concrete, which reflects this glare. Rain makes the walkways slippery at times, as does snow and ice. Any rises or ledges that occur in the walkway should be clearly marked in a contrasting value or intensity of color to the walkway surface.

Doors present a variety of problems at entrance ways into buildings. There is an abundant use of glass doors in nursing homes, which seems to be a spinoff from other commercial construction. Perception of precisely where the door is in relation to the position of the user is made difficult by this transparent, shiny, and reflective surface. These doors are also very heavy and utilize hinging systems—self-closing types—that impede ease of use by the elderly. Some use is being made of power actuated doors, which are triggered by foot pressure, similar to the doors found in super-markets and airports. This necessitates two-door systems to expedite entrance and egress if the doors are swinging hinged types. Here again, a perilous situation exists whereby an elderly person using the wrong door, triggered by someone using the right door can be knocked down and seriously injured. These types of doors must be clearly marked with appropriate graphics that can be seen and identified under a variety of lighting conditions, or access to the wrong door must be made impossible through design detailing (see Figure 59).

The problem of the powered door on swinging hinges can be alleviated by the use of powered sliding doors, which can be approached from either side without imperiling the user on the other side. These systems are expensive and fall into disrepair far more frequently than nonpowered doorways.

If the doors are glass, it is important to frame or otherwise mark the surface of the door in a non-reflective material or paint so that its position can be perceived easily. Pressure needed to open the door should not be excessive and should be constant, so that the door does not suddenly lunge open and cause a fall.

The interior of the entrance way is an extremely important place for both the visitor and the patient-resident entering the first time, using this space constantly, and using it as a lounging area. One neglected facet of its design is proper lighting control. Many entranceways are quite dark, and the shift from inside to outside, or vice versa, is very pro-nounced. Once again, this is an accident-inducing problem. Although excessive glazing will render a condition of excessive glare, there should be con-trolled exterior light—perhaps transluscent panels—penetrating the space so that an effective transition for the eyes is made.

In some nursing homes there is an effort made to discourage use of the entrance way or lobby by the patient–residents who reside there. Yet this is a heavily traveled area and very attractive to those who enjoy sitting and watching activity. The same requirements are applicable for the lobby space as a lounge bay in the corridor-neighborhood concept. The entrance area may or may not be a part of the corridor neigh-borhood, but the activity present will draw some of the patient–residents there.

Another important consideration in the design of this space is the use of directional and visual markers to expedite the finding of locations within the facility. The posting of any directory should be prominent. Use of large-alphabet type faces and numerical symbols with color coding related to specific wings or parts of the facility should be the predominant method of quickly relating the user to any specific part of the building plan. The plan of the building layout itself should be visually displayed and marked according to the system of coding. For those with impaired sight, the texture- or shape-coding system employed through-out the building should be presented so that this process of identification can be learned and used.

It may be necessary as well as an interesting idea to have patient–residents or volunteers engaged near the directory who can assist others in the use of the direc-tory—especially sight-impaired persons—and also expedite the quick location of areas in the building. In this way, it would not be necessary to learn an entire and somewhat complicated system to visit one part of the building.

It is also extremely important to consider the impression created by the entrance area in relationship to the rest of the facility. Frequently, the entrance way is used to present a false facade for a facility. The entrance area is made especially attractive to create an impression of the facility itself. Many visitors to a given facility may never go beyond the entrance way itself; the impression they derive at that point is the only impression they have. However, this reliance upon first impressions works to the adverse when a visitor or a prospective client penetrates space beyond the entrance area. The real nature of the facility shows very quickly, and questions arise about administra-tion and staff who create false facades in the physical environment; what about the delivery of health ser-

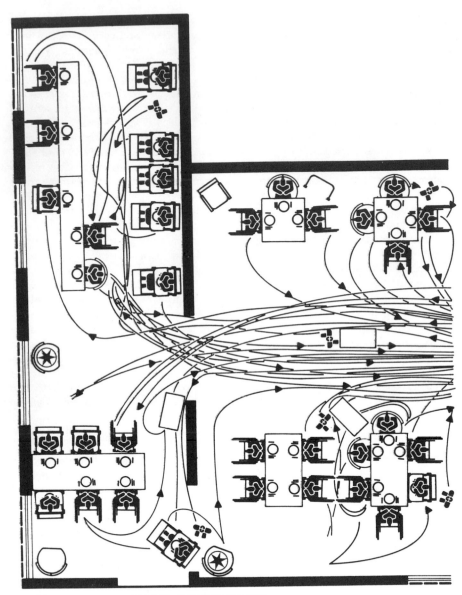

42-039-163 Dining Room 12:10-1:07; 42-040-163 12:10-12:55

FIGURE 53 (*above and right*)

Large dining room space. Large central dining facilities may very well be outmoded with new food service techniques. However, the importance of the dining room cannot be understated because it houses one activity that is highly therapeutic and valued by the patient–residents. A single large dining space is furnished with six-place tables arranged in a back-to-back configuration. This makes ingress and egress from the space and the tables difficult. The four-place table provides better accessibility and also fewer problems regarding interaction with companions.

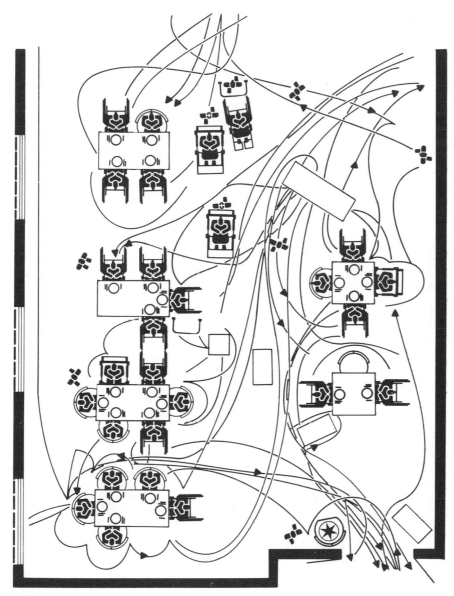

42-O4I-I63 Dining Room 12:2O-12:53

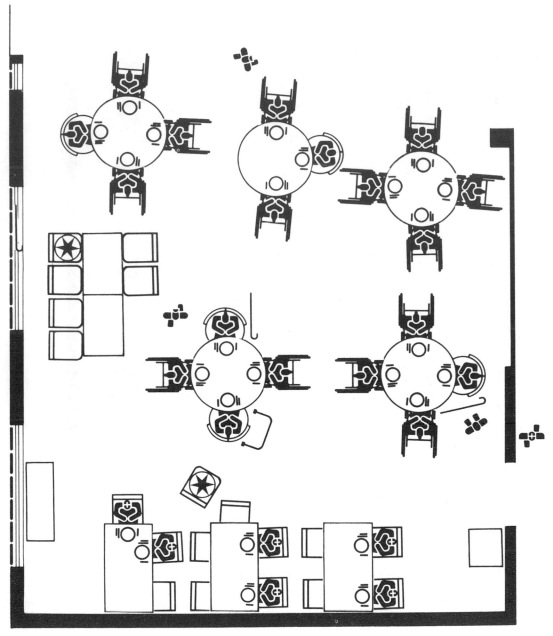

22-011-263 Dining Room 12:25-1:17

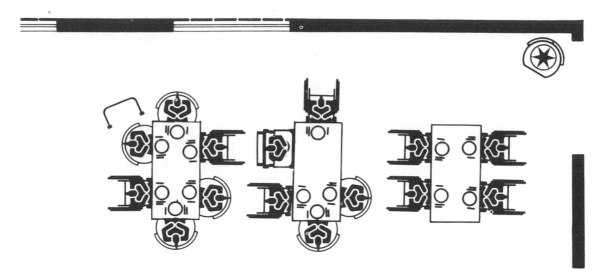

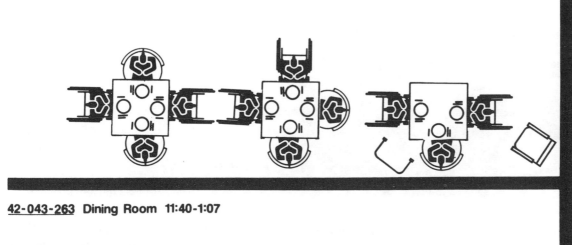

42-043-263 Dining Room 11:40-1:07

FIGURE 54 (*left and above*)
Dining rooms with open access. The two alternatives to the problem of handling the traffic in dining rooms are represented here. Either four-place tables must be used throughout with access from any side (the round shape also facilitates this approach), or there must be adequate aisle width for maneuvering the ambulatory devices.

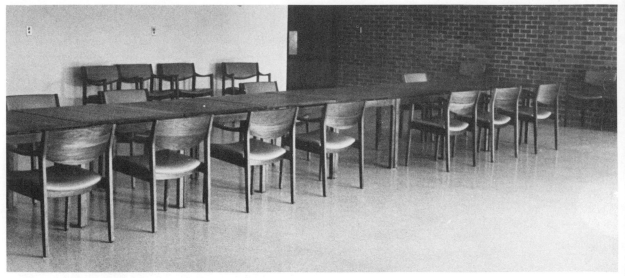

FIGURE 55
Dining room furnishings with side-to-side interaction problems. (Photo: John Kelsey and Robert Steinbugler.)

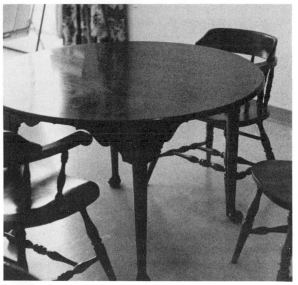

FIGURE 56
Dining room chair that cannot penetrate beneath the table apron. (Photo: John Kelsey and Robert Steinbugler.)

vices and what people are being told about it during a visit?

There should be no deviation in the esthetics from the entrance to any other portion of the facility. There should be no change in atmosphere, no abrupt

sense of disparity. There should be the same consideration given to the farthest portion from the entrance as to the entrance itself; and the character, quality, esthetics, and atmosphere of the entrance should be inviting and intriguing.

FIGURE 57

Bathroom studies. It is necessary to provide grip rails around both sides of the toilet. There is a high incidence of paralysis on one side of the body among patient–resident populations. One grip rail provides a transfer assist to those who either have no loss of strength or have diminished strength on the side away from the grip rail. Furthermore, the rails should provide for a vertical thrust of strength and not an extension outward away from the center of gravity of the torso. (Photo: John Kelsey and Robert Steinbugler.)

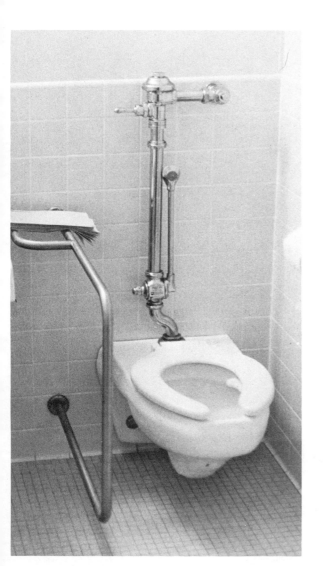

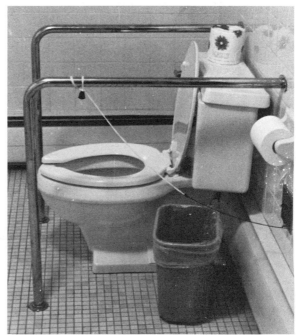

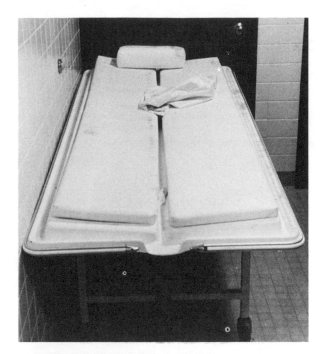

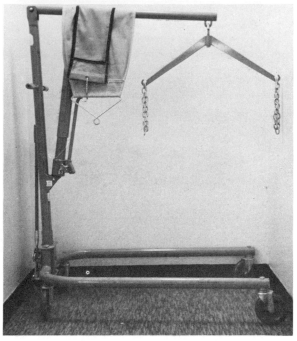

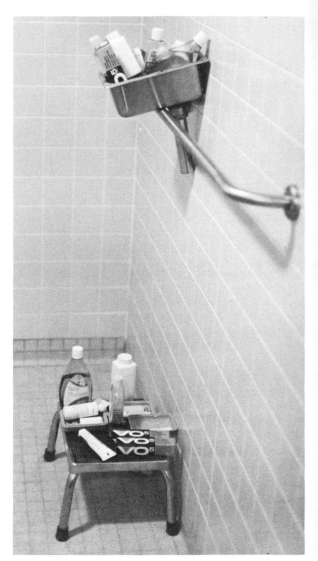

OUTSIDE AREAS

The use and the meaning of the outside grounds, decks, or walkways are significant in the design of the facility. Frequently, the procedure and method of access is so complex and removed from the patient-resident that very little exposure to the outside, if any, is received at all (see Figure 8). One problem is that the only solution employed in most architecture is to make a pronounced difference, if not barrier, between inside and outside. In fact, in a large majority of facilities there is access to the outside only through the main entrance of the building. Other exits are merely fire or emergency exits used only after complex latching mechanisms are triggered and alarm systems are set off.

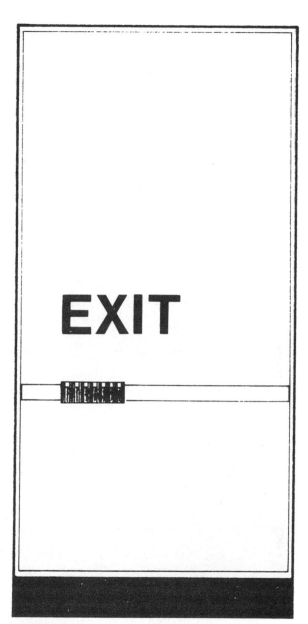

FIGURE 58 (*left*)

Bathroom studies: storage problems. These three photographs show the problem of storing both personal effects of patients and the devices necessary for effective cleaning, transfer, and therapy (examining functions). Typically, there is a degree of "afterthought" when it comes to integrating the tools and devices necessary for proper care in the bathroom area. (Photo Credit: John Kelsey and Robert Steinbugler.)

FIGURE 59

Doorways. Doors should be clearly and boldly marked for their purpose. Handles should be orientated away from the hinge pins of the door, indicating the opening side and greatest leverage. Handles should be elongated rails rather than either discs or cylinders. The graphics on the door glass should indicate the surface so as not to confuse the visually impared user.

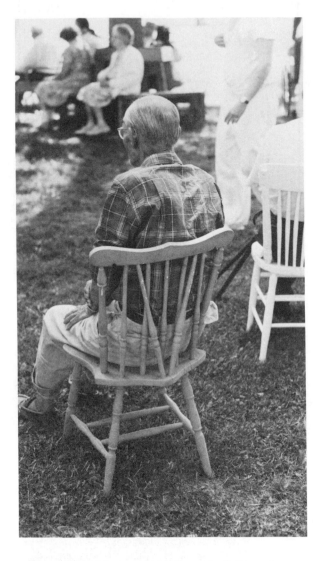

FIGURE 60

Outside activity. It is important to program outside activities into the routine for the elderly who reside in the institutional setting. It is equally important to provide amenities in keeping with the setting and safe for patient-resident use. One of the most important assets of the old home and farm arrangement was that the activities grew directly out of the very nature of the setting, and there were things to do that the elderly who resided therein had done all their lives. Many of those settings were inefficient and provided very poor living conditions. A few, like this home and farm in upstate New York, were well run and provided lessons about institutionalization that have not been learned by more contemporary facility planners and administrators. (Photo: John Kelsey and Robert Steinbugler.)

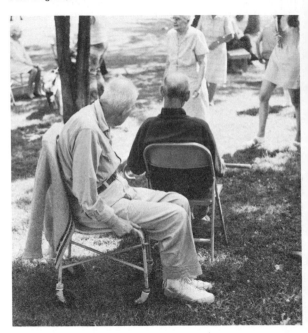

There should be access to the out-of-doors, to sunshine and fresh air, without having to exit the facility (see Figure 60). Thus there should be areas accessible to the outside environment from the corridor neighborhood (Figures 11 and 14).

Many architectural devices could be employed to provide this kind of exposure without penetrating beyond the physical facility itself. Solaria can be modified to permit external environmental exposure when the weather and season permit. The roofing system could extend beyond the building support walls to provide a shroud bounded by an external glass wall with exposure on two ends to permit airflow. Obviously, the grounds beyond should be visually stimulating or there should be a view of activity in the surrounding neighborhood or community. Often the side of the building where traffic predominates is more preferable to patient-residents

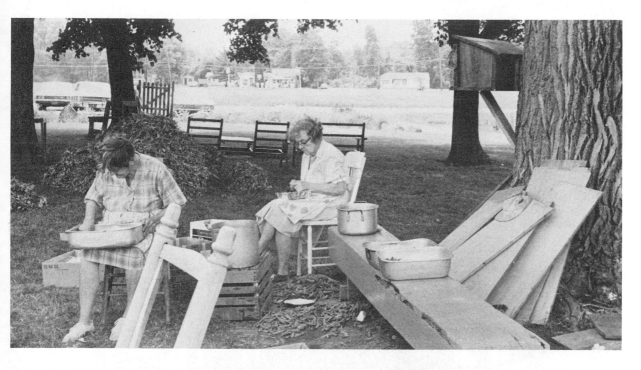

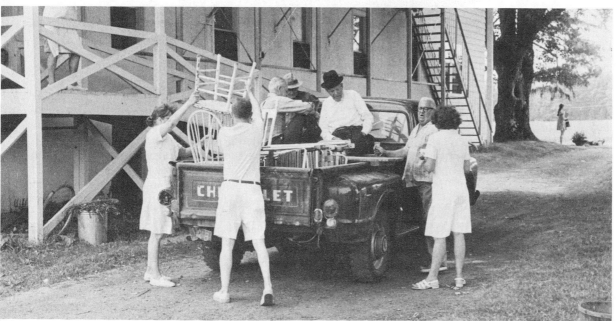

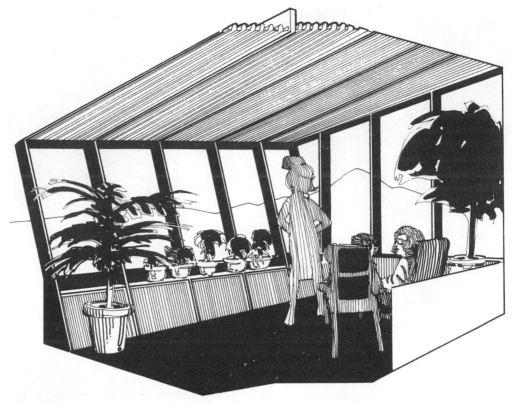

FIGURE 61
Outside areas. There is a need for protected outside areas that provide for sitting, socialization, and activity, with shrouding to reduce glare and weather-control baffles. These areas should be multifunctional and very accessible.

than the more passive or bucolic side of the building (Figure 35).

It is important as well to provide a visual screen to reduce exposure to glare, with adequate seating for rest, relaxation, and retreat. Frequently, the outside areas of a facility are not at all utilized even though exposure is readily accessible because the glare is very bothersome.

Ganged, in-line seating should be avoided in protected areas as well as on the grounds of a facility. The outdoor furniture should be suitable for no more than two person use, and each side should be equipped with arms for ease of entrance and egress. Seating should be arranged so that there is a clear

view of activity and/or conversational groupings are promoted (Figure 61).

Where there are grounds attached to a facility, the plantings or gardens should either be unprotected or high 30-inch barriers used to prevent trampling. Many facilities use low barriers, frequently in concrete, to edge a flower garden. It is more preferable that a petunia be trampled than an aging person be tripped and injured by a low barrier that can go unseen in the glare and harsh outside natural lighting (Figure 62).

The construction of walkways and ramps is often a problem in nursing home construction. As the supporting ground beneath concrete shifts over time,

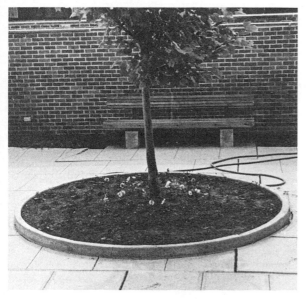

FIGURE 62
Outdoor flower bed. Unfortunately, more attention was given to the protection of the flowers in this outdoor garden than to the safety of the elderly infirm who use this outside area. It would be difficult for an older person with vision problems to see the edge of this flower bed. The design is potentially very hazardous. (Photo: John Kelsey and Robert Steinbugler.)

the cement will lift at the edge and present a definite hazard to the ambulatory patient–resident. These distortions in the walking surface should be watched for and guarded against constantly. The problem can be avoided to a degree by using other materials to surface walks. However, nothing will withstand wear and tear over time as well as the poured concrete surface.

Ramps are one of the more unsuccessful devices to employ within a facility. Used to some degree in the interiors of buildings as well as the outside, the ramp is an impediment to the ambulatory because of the profound change in the walking gait of the elderly. The erect, off-balance, shuffling movement becomes extraordinarily difficult even when the degree of rise is slight. Exterior ramps usually are designed with a severe degree or angle of rise be-

cause slight angles mean a long expanse of ramp to connect level changes. Many of these ramps are not usable without assistance. There is also little possibility that a wheelchair-bound semiambulatory patient–resident can use exterior ramps without assistance either. Loss of control of a wheelchair on an exterior ramp can mean a very serious accident.

In summary, the ramp is probably not the answer for level changes on either the exterior or within the interior of a facility for the aging. The facility itself must be designed so that level changes without the use of elevators are minimized if not excluded.

To summarize this chapter very briefly, the major thesis is that there should be a shift away from isolated spaces delegated to specific functions within the facility to a facility model in which the functions are accommodated within more generalized spaces more proximate to the location of the patient–resident. This concept is embodied in the corridor neighborhood. In addition, the social, recreational, activity, and retreat functions attributable to the lounge and general activity spaces should be shifted to the patient–resident room, the corridor outside of the room, and more personalized lounge and dining spaces off the corridor.

There must be a real attempt to build in residency in the physical environment. This quality has been largely neglected in order to heighten the delivery of health care—in essence, making the nursing home atmosphere a kind of hospital. This is not appropriate to the kind of rehabilitation necessary to promote real rebuilding of the patient–resident who has sustained a trauma and is in a regressive or deterioration stage of life physiologically. There should be a sense of residency in these specialized environments to provide a continuity between the temporary status in the health care environment and the home environment. Abrupt changes or restrictions upon the patient–resident cause feelings of anxiety and apprehension, which do not promote healing but do promote further deterioration and the acquisition of new symptoms.

The sense of residency is largely dependent upon how quickly a patient–resident can be drawn into the program and activities that are a part of his or her rehabilitation. Therefore, the physical environment must be designed to maximize accessibility to activity, both from the standpoint of being passively engaged and actively engaged.

The amount of time any given patient–resident spends as the recipient of health care services is a small fraction of his or her total time. Yet the whole facility at present is designed around this delivery, and minimal attention is given to accommodating this person during the majority of the residency. There should be a reversal of this design direction so that the health care nature of the facility is subdued and plays a supportive role to the other aspects of the facility program.

REFERENCES

Goldsmith, Selwyn, *Designing for the Disabled*. London: Royal Institute of British Architects, 1967.

Kieselbach, Richard, and Richard Hatch. "Vision and Lighting at First Community Village." In *First Community Village Report*, Joseph A. Koncelik (ed.). Unpublished Manuscript. Columbus, O.: Department of Industrial Design, Ohio State University, 1975.

Kira, Alexander. *The Bathroom: Criteria for Design.* Ithaca, N.Y.: Cornell University, Center for Housing and Environmental Studies, 1966.

Koncelik, Joseph A., Edward Ostrander, and Lorraine H. Snyder. *The Relationship of the Physical Environment in 6 Extended Care Facilities to the Behavior of Their Resident Aging People.* Research Report No. 103. Ithaca, N.Y.: Department of Design and Environmental Analysis, College of Human Ecology, Cornell University, 1972.

Parsons, Henry M. "The Bedroom." *Human Factors*, 14, no. 5 (1972), pp. 421–450.

President's Committee on Employment of the Handicapped. Recommendations of the Subcommittee on Barrier Free Design, Pamphlet ANSI Standard 117.1, *Making Buildings Accessible and Usable by the Physically Handicapped.* Washington, D.C.: Superintendent of Documents, 1971.

Progner, Jean W. "The Sociologist and the Designer Can Be Friends." *Design and Environment* (Spring 1971). New York: R. C. Publications.

Snyder, Lorraine H., E. Ostrander, and J. A. Koncelik. *The New Nursing Home*, Conference Proceedings. Ithaca, N.Y.: Cornell University, College of Human Ecology, mimeographed report, June 1973, pp. 37–47.

RECOMMENDATIONS FOR SEATING, FURNISHINGS, AND BEDS

SEATING

Where people sit and what they sit on is perhaps the most significant design problem in the design of a nursing home facility outside of the specific configuration of spaces the patient-resident uses. In fact, for some of the more severely disabled occupants of a nursing home, the device in which they are seated becomes their environment; the other surroundings become effectively meaningless. There are seven general problems affecting the range of types of seating devices used in a nursing home:

1. Ambulatory status of the patient-resident.
2. General physiological problems associated with seating and seated position.
3. Seated durations and posture.
4. Function of the specific seating type.
5. Research and development of new seating.
6. Applications of new available technology.
7. Problems in manufacturing and distribution.

Ambulatory Status of the Patient-Resident

Interestingly enough, one neglected prerequisite in furnishing a nursing home is determining the projected ambulatory status of the population of clients who will reside in the home. This is readily apparent when even the casual observer enters a nursing home and sees how much stationary furnishing is not being used on most occasions. Reference has already been made in the planning chapter to the effect of this on space and choice of seating. In many nursing homes, if the appropriate seating was chosen on the basis of ambulatory status, the general feel of most spaces would be entirely different—sparse or empty. In this lies the problem. Given a particular room, the temptation is to locate chairs around the space in pleasant arrangements.

Unfortunately, these arrangements are often based upon the conceptions of either design staffs or administrators, which relate to conversations among younger ambulatory people. In other words, the furnishings selected are often inappropriate for non-ambulatory people, and the distances between furnishings and the number of furnishings (chairs) are frequently both too great.

Where research has been conducted tracing the development of a given facility, it has been shown that one very important problem is the retention of design consultation throughout the actual design process. All too frequently, the architect or interior designer is not given the opportunity to advise on the selection of furnishings or the interior decor. This is almost tragic because there are so many functional considerations concerning human factors, anthropometrics, and behavioral requirements that should enter the total picture of design at this level. For the most part, someone who is an administrator or part of the staff of a facility is usually placed in charge of "buying" the furnishings, and the most important criterion becomes economics at the point of purchase. Often, the most economical choice at the point of purchase is the least economical choice as a useful piece of goods or as a durable commodity.

Generally, if an administrator wishes to have his or her office designed a certain way there is no harm in the administrator doing the design or selection of furnishings. Perhaps no one is more qualified to select equipment for an occupational therapy area or for a physiotherapy area than the professionals who are engaged in that activity. This does not mean that the expertise they have been trained for is transferable to all other areas of interior design.

Many architectural firms have excellent interior design services within their own organization, or they are able to refer their clients to reputable interior design firms that have the capability to deal with the special problems of nursing home interiors. Administrators with the best intentions simply cannot be so equipped to deal with the large number of criteria essential in the buying and selection decisions. This does not mean that administrators should not enter this process. It is extremely important that the staff or personnel who will be making replacement purchases and refurbishing decisions enter into these design decisions and participate with the designers so that there is mutuality and unanimity with regard to the choice of furnishings.

Another acute problem in the selection process is that the designer who produces designs for geriatric furniture does not have direct contact with the problems and people who will be using his designs. This situation is complicated by the fact that very few pieces of furniture are ever really designed by professional designers. There are over 5000 furniture manufacturers in the United States, but only about 25

firms either employ outside designers or have designers on staff.

In other words, the problem of getting appropriate seating and furnishings for a nursing home is complicated by the lack of availability of well-designed pieces in the first place and the reluctance on the part of the manufacturers—or their inability—to finance design development, second.

Between 30 and 70 percent of the population in the nursing home (on the average 50 percent) will be confined to either wheelchairs or mobile geriatric chairs. This means that a large segment of the population will not be using stationary furnishings. Such furnishings are likely to impede their free use of space if excessive amounts are purchased for any given space in the nursing home that the user gains access to. For the most part, nonambulatory patient-residents will bring their mobile chairs to the spaces they frequent and will not transfer or be transferred to stationary furnishings.

One of the most important developments in this regard, if this hypothesis is accepted as a premise for design, is that the stationary geriatric chair, produced in fairly large quantities, is essentially functionless in a nursing home where the staff does not transfer nonambulatory patients to stationary seating. The slick and untextured vinyl to promote ease of cleaning after incontinence and the spread of the base of legs to provide a stable surface for transfer are criteria applied to a seating type that is largely dysfunctional in a large majority of nursing homes. As will be shown in the section on function of the specific seating type, these criteria are not based upon the real nature of the requirements of the population. Generally, incontinence is related to three factors which affect seating: (1) ambulatory status—the more incontinent population is nonambulatory, (2) incontinence is a form of very effective protest by a population offended by the care they are receiving and the stiff hierarchy of social relationships in the nursing home, (3) and extreme use of "management" drugs, which have a long-term effect on the physiology, including incontinence. For some peculiar reason (or very understandable reasons depending on point of view), European countries that have industries manufacturing geriatric chairs do not use vinyl trim on the surfaces of their products. They use fabrics, and frequently the seating is contoured and pleated. This either shows a profound sense and understanding of the situation regarding the nature of incontinence among the elderly, or they are producing seating in almost complete disregard for the problems the elderly present to designers.

There is a pressing need to investigate more fully the relationship between loss of ambulatory status—a significant level of deterioration in physical health of the aging patient–resident—and incontinence. Furthermore, research on this relationship would provide more definite evidence to support or refute what seems to be a very improper set of design criteria associated with the wrong population and the assumption that incontinence is purely a physiological problem.

It is not unusual for patient–residents in wheelchairs or those partially or fully ambulatory to associate advanced levels of illness to patient–residents who must use the mobile geriatric chair. Even though some in this nonambulatory population are very alert, communicative, and otherwise capable, they become associated with senility and advanced physiological problems by virtue of their ambulatory status. It is, in fact, a strange form of prejudice, which is unjustified in many cases.

The very nature of the geriatric chair, its configuration, differences from other seating, restraint characteristics, and qualities implying incapacitation of the user help classify that user as incompetent. The seating device, then, is responsible for further isolation and perjorative judgments from staff and fellow patient–residents (Figures 63 and 69).

There must be new design development to create a totally different set of mobile seating devices for the nursing home. There is no question that problems associated with ambulatory status have been interpreted wrongly, and the interpretations made are exacerbating unresolved problems.

General Physiological Problems Associated with Seating and the Seated Position

One critical factor in the design of all seating, regardless of population ages and physiological status, is that approximately 60 percent of the load of the body rests or is supported on the ischial tuberosities at the base of the hip bone. This is a concentration of load on two protuberances in the bone structure, which are compressing the tissue beneath. Essentially, then, total comfort is greatly dependent upon how well the weight or load of the torso is supported, suspended, and dissipated at these points (Figure 64).

The aging person has substantially less fatty and muscle tissue between the ischial tuberosities and the chair surface. Thus, because there is less capacity to disperse the load through the tissues of the body itself and greater compression of the existing tissues, discomfort or pain happens more quickly (Figure 64).

The problem of ease of entrance and egress from stationary seating for the ambulatory and semiambulatory (with walkers and canes) is an important consideration, which has received much attention. The healthy and younger person is able to move the heel of the foot backward under the surface of the chair more proximate to the line of the center of gravity, lifting away from the seat surface through the power of the leg muscles alone. The elderly person is not able to perform the egress function in this manner. Gradually, the older person becomes ever more reliant upon the grip of the hand on an arm of a chair and the pull of the arm muscles to egress a chair (Figures 63 and 64).

Entrance and egress for the mobile are also affected by the height of the seat platform from the floor and the tilt or angle backward off the horizontal of the platform. The lower the platform, the lower the center of gravity is seated in the chair, and the harder it is for the older person to extract himself or herself from the chair. The lower the platform, the greater the distance necessary for the leg muscles to raise the torso vertically. Also, the knee angle assumes an acute angle relationship between the upper and lower leg. For many elderly, exaggerated acute angles are impossible and for most, very difficult. Frequently, the observer will see an elderly person seated in a low chair thrust his or her legs to an open angle with the lower legs forward. Another part of the problem is that, when a chair is low, the elderly person will not be able to lower his or her weight into a chair beyond a certain point. Frequently, they will reach a point where

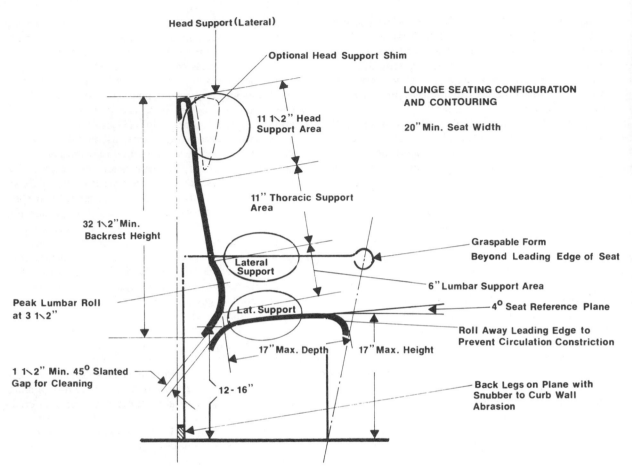

Head Support (Lateral)

Optional Head Support Shim

LOUNGE SEATING CONFIGURATION
AND CONTOURING

20" Min. Seat Width

11 1\2" Head
Support Area

11" Thoracic Support
Area

32 1\2" Min.
Backrest Height

Graspable Form
Beyond Leading Edge of Seat

Lateral
Support

6" Lumbar Support Area

Peak Lumbar Roll
at 3 1\2"

4° Seat Reference Plane

Lat. Support

Roll Away Leading Edge to
Prevent Circulation Constriction

17" Max. Depth   17" Max. Height

1 1\2" Min. 45° Slanted
Gap for Cleaning

Back Legs on Plane with
Snubber to Curb Wall
Abrasion

12 - 16"

FIGURE 63
Seat design criteria.

they drop their weight to the surface of the chair (Figure 64).

If the angle off the horizontal of the platform is too excessive, it will prevent easy egress of the chair, as well as promote the dropping of the weight at entry because of the lower area to the rear of the platform. The combination of deflection of trim materials and angle off horizontal are two critical design considerations with regard to promoting ease of egress when there is less general muscular strength and flexibility at the joints.

Another serious physiological consideration is that of the roll of the spine at the shoulders. Much of the seating devised for the elderly tapers away at the shoulders and does not afford proper support. There should be a change of angle, undetermined without further seating research and development, to accommodate this important consideration. The spine and back are also less flexible. There is less adaptive capacity to assume a range of postures to conform to a variety of seating (Figure 64).

The elderly will generally use the back supports in most seating. Although this seems an obvious criterion for all seating, it is a fundamental and singularly

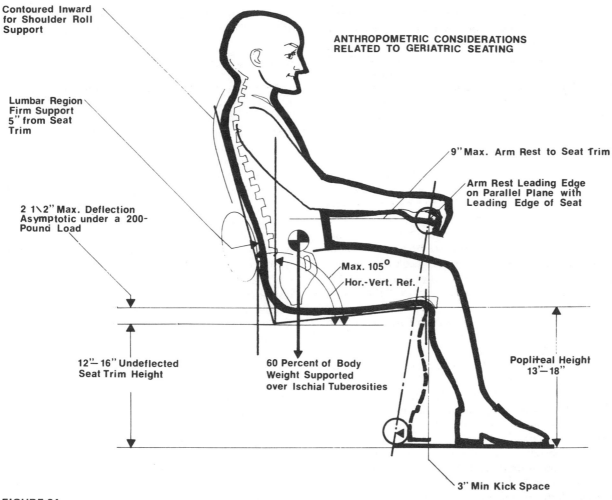

Contoured Inward
for Shoulder Roll
Support

ANTHROPOMETRIC CONSIDERATIONS
RELATED TO GERIATRIC SEATING

Lumbar Region
Firm Support
5" from Seat
Trim

9" Max. Arm Rest to Seat Trim

Arm Rest Leading Edge
on Parallel Plane with
Leading Edge of Seat

2 1\2" Max. Deflection
Asymptotic under a 200-
Pound Load

Max. 105°
Hor.-Vert. Ref.

12"—16" Undeflected
Seat Trim Height

60 Percent of Body
Weight Supported
over Ischial Tuberosities

Popliteal Height
13"—18"

3" Min Kick Space

FIGURE 64
Anthropometric and body position criteria.

important criterion in the design of functional seating, such as dining seating. Since the back support will be used over a long period of time, the relationship of distance between chair back and table surface is extremely important. When an arm is not able to penetrate beneath the surface of a table, the distance between back support and edge of table is too excessive for the eating function to be performed satisfactorily. Younger people will lean forward in their chairs and accommodate to an unsatisfactory situation, but the elderly user of this type of seating cannot do this easily or for any length of time (Figure 64).

Muscle fatigue, general muscle capacity and strength in compression of tissue, support of weight on the spinal column, and flexibility and rotation of the pelvis (Figure 64) are all important problems to be dealt with in all seating design, and especially in designs for the elderly. There are, however, two other physiological considerations that are more important in seating design for the elderly than for other age groups: (1) effects upon circulation and (2) effects upon respiration. Because of the durations and posture of the person in the chair, there is or can be constrictions of circulation and respiration owing to the assumed angularities of the body and pressures exerted upon critical areas by the chair surfaces (Figure 64).

It has been argued by many who have studied seating for the elderly that the height of the leading edge of the seat platform should be about 17 or 18 inches from the floor (Laging, 1972). Some have argued that the greater the height, the better the conditions of entrance and egress. For the shorter elderly person, those under 5 feet 4 inches in height, a critical factor is the pressure exerted under the knee by the leading edge of the platform compressing veins and arteries and shutting off blood supply, after even short durations of seated time.

It should be kept in mind that the highest proportion of client patient–residents in the nursing home are women. Their height range is from 4 feet 7 inches to 5 feet 4½ inches (90 percent of the population from 75 to 79 years of age). This population also has a popliteal height of from 13½ inches to approximately 17 inches. This means that the height of the chair seat platform at the leading edge should not exceed 17 inches, and probably should be lower in order to accommodate the largest majority of the elderly users without causing excessive pressure beneath the knee to the unprotected veins and arteries. Higher platform heights will result in dangling feet and a curious numbness in the lower extremities after even a relatively short seated time (Figure 63).

Respiration will become affected adversely if the angle between the upper torso and the upper legs is constricted and held without change for any length of time. Because of the roll of the spine forward and the lift of the seat platform at the leading edge, this problem can become acute, especially when the durations of seated time become long. Although there is no design revelation that will change this condition, it is important for the designer to be aware of this problem if he is not going to exacerbate it by constricting the open angle of the seat.

Seated Durations and Posture

Reference has been made to the durations of time an aging person occupies a chair and also the relevance of this time as it affects posture. Observations have revealed that ambulatory elderly in nursing homes occupy chairs for as long as six hours without moving from them. In some cases ambulatory patient-residents of extended care facilities have been observed to stay seated for eight hours. Most astounding of all, nonambulatory patient-residents have been observed to occupy their mobile geriatric chairs or wheelchairs for as long as twelve hours. Observations of this kind were made during the research conducted by Koncelik, Ostrander, and Snyder (1972).

It seems fruitless to recommend that patient-residents be moved out of chairs or transferred more frequently. The nonambulatory patient–resident has two possible behaviors in this regard: lying down and sitting up. Also, the staff other than nursing—and frequently the nurses as well—are engaged for the greater part of the day in moving people about, transferring patient-residents from one position to another, and, in general, repositioning patient-residents.

The problem of long seated durations in the nursing home must be approached and solved through the design of seating, because there is no foreseeable alternative. The key questions are, then, what are the major considerations related to long periods of seated time, and how can the problems presented be approached through design?

One of the most serious results of this phenomenon are decubitus ulcers because of the prolonged pressure on the buttocks tissue. The person who must sit for long periods is actually attempting to avoid decubitus spreading over a greater portion of his or her body by not lying down all day in bed. One of the most important changes that should be made in the design of mobile geriatric chairs, especially in this regard, is the rejection of rigid platform bases and the use of spring bases, especially rubber diaphragms and webbing. Most mobile geriatric chair

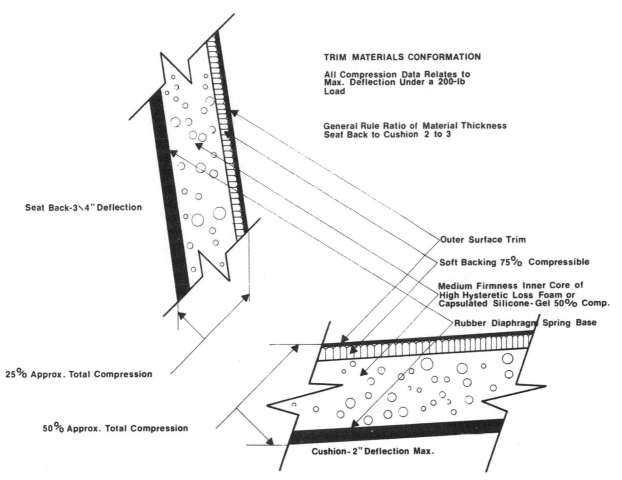

TRIM MATERIALS CONFORMATION

All Compression Data Relates to Max. Deflection Under a 200-lb Load

General Rule Ratio of Material Thickness Seat Back to Cushion 2 to 3

Seat Back-3\4" Deflection

25% Approx. Total Compression

50% Approx. Total Compression

Outer Surface Trim

Soft Backing 75% Compressible

Medium Firmness Inner Core of High Hysteretic Loss Foam or Capsulated Silicone-Gel 50% Comp.

Rubber Diaphragm Spring Base

Cushion-2" Deflection Max.

FIGURE 65
Seat suspension criteria.

platforms "bottom" or reach a deflection point where there is no possible further deflection left in the suspension media. This causes even greater pressure to be exerted upon the ischial tuberosities and the tissue beneath them. Making use of a full suspension system in the seat base instead of only a partial seating suspension system should go a long way to help solve this problem (Figure 65).

Aside from the potential of a full suspension media incorporated in mobile geriatric chairs, other tech-

nological innovations could be applied to this type and other types of institutional seating, such as the use of silicone gel cushions and deep foam molding for seat platforms.

Figures 66–70 show geriatric chairs and some of the problems discussed.

Another aspect of long durations in one seating device is support and restraint from falling or sliding from the chair. Often, the elderly who occupy a chair for an extended period of time fall asleep. As

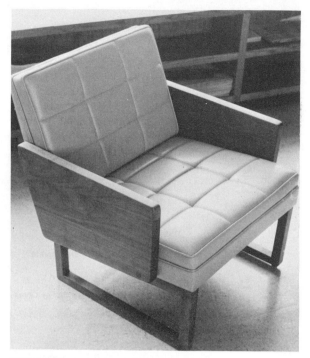

FIGURE 66
Nongeriatric chair in the nursing home setting. This chair has been shown in earlier photographs and may be an extremely good piece of furniture—but not in the nursing home. The leading edge is too low and the arms do not extend forward enough to provide leverage to move the torso center of gravity up and out during egress. The backrest is too low to provide adequate support to the thoracic region of the back as well as to the shoulders. (Photo: John Kelsey and Robert Steinbugler.)

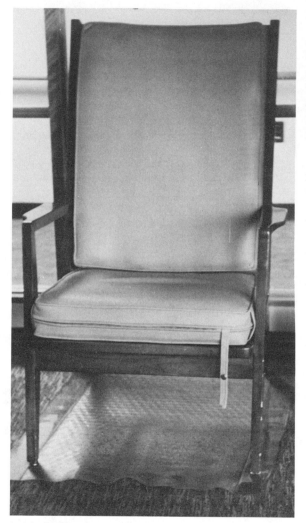

FIGURE 67
Geriatric chair in the nursing home setting. Although the dimensions of this chair are more suitable for its intended purpose, it still does not provide lateral support for the sleeping patient–resident nor is the backrest properly contoured. There is obviously a great concern for the need to protect against incontinence. Yet, the question of whether this problem should be rectified in the lounge and in chair design or through the provision of more strategically placed bathrooms is unanswered, primarily because so few nursing homes provide a bathroom near lounges! (Photo: John Kelsey and Robert Steinbugler.)

they do, they tend to move either forward or to the side and slip from the chair. It is not impossible to have a very incapacitated patient–resident slide over the side of a chair, even over an armrest. Side support and head supports on either side or one side of the chair are necessary appointments in the development of these furnishings. Often referred to as wings, these devices may extend the full length of the back of the chair or be positioned only at the top leading edge. Likewise, the armrest is an important partial restraint, and so would be side contouring of the seat platform and the seat back cushion (Figure 64).

There is a great deal of difference between the partial restraint needed for support while sitting and the full restraint meant to secure a patient–resident in a chair. This is the most odious spectacle the observer confronts in the nursing home: people tied to chairs. Patient–residents being restrained in beds seem more understandable than this aspect of nursing home life. In this frame of reference, the duration in a chair as a result of choice becomes duration as a result of mandate. This seems to result from a prevailing fear on the part of many staff that certain patient–residents will wander about and hurt themselves through a fall or other mishap. There are special people who need to be restrained lest they do injury to themselves. However, it is possible to restrain a patient through chair design. A tilting chair with high leading edge might be just as effective as tying people down.

The designer must confront this problem forthrightly and with understanding. Unfortunately, the devices usually contrived to keep people in one place are makeshift and sometimes dangerous. Often called "bellybands," a variety of devices are used to tie down patient–residents who might wander. There have been examples of patient–residents slipping out of their restraint and catching themselves on it under the chin and at the throat.

It is interesting that most mobile geriatric chairs, and other versions as well, are equipped with demountable trays which serve as eating surfaces or general-use surfaces. These can be effective restraint devices if they are properly designed and used. The surround of the chair, depth of the cushioning, angle of the leading edge, and other characteristics of the design could be so articulated that they become the effective restraint.

The greater share of human factors and anthropometric data on seated posture emphasizes the effect of seated angles (angles assumed because of the angles of the seat) on the position of the body. This information treats the human torso as if it were completely pliant and could assume any angle according to the design of the chair. There are two factors involved in seated posture: (1) the assumed seated angles and (2) the physiological pliance of the human being who is seated. Given any chair, there will be a wide variance between angles, position of the body, roll of the pelvis, and distribution of weight according to the relationship of both factors (1) and (2). A set of seated angle relationships will change radically depending on the seated penetration of one person compared with another. A thin person under 150 pounds might sink into the seat cushion to a greater depth than a 200-pound person whose weight is dispersed over a wider surface area on the cushion. For one person, the seated angles might be quite severe and for the other, quite open and obtuse. Obviously, working with a set of static seated angles is not totally satisfactory. The designer must consider the configuration of the design and the combination of specific materials employed in order to achieve seating that is suitable for the widest range of people.

The way in which seat configurations have been determined in the automotive industry occurs in essentially three phases. First, a large assembly of data was collected on the position of the skeletal frame in a variety of seated positions. This information was used to generate a posterior contour for three percentile groups among the total population: the fifth percentile, the fiftieth percentile, and the ninetieth percentile. The second phase was the design and limited manufacture of both two- and three-dimensional manikins to be used in both the development and evaluation of seating. The third phase was the development of a uniform procedure to be used in the design and development of all seating for American automobiles, so that all seating could meet uniform standards and be checked independently by any manufacturer.

Today, the automotive industry both in America and abroad has an internal technology of seating design unparalleled by any other industry or independent testing body. This industry also has an accumulation of knowledge about seating design, conformation of materials, and dynamic testing that can be considered a science of seat design.

Although the furniture manufacturing industry is not nearly as organized and as powerful as the automotive industry, there must be uniform standards created and the same degree, if not a greater degree, of intensity applied to learning more about the dynamics of seating and posture in seated durations. A chair might conform exceptionally well to the available standards of angularities and dimensions currently used in the design of "static" seating (seating that is not used as a supportive platform in vehicles). However, the conformation of materials, the densities, differences of thicknesses, and deflections in the materials, might produce entirely inappropriate angularities in posture. This is essentially the state of the art today in seating design.

An interesting unpublished paper by Michael French (1975) contains the basic beginning steps for generating this technology. His experiments in 1973 and 1974 in determining differences in seated posture according to materials use and angularities of the seat frame were not totally successful but were extremely provocative as a beginning in the long process of creating the needed information useful in putting together the first phase of a technology and set of standards. French designed and built a frame and support mechanism that varied in angular relationship. Through a right-angle brace with movable probes, he was able to determine the rough contour of the seated profile or the posterior of a seated elderly person in his test device. French measured the posterior of over 20 aged patient-residents in the nursing section of a retirement community.

Although his results were inconclusive, his experiments clearly demonstrate that work of this kind *can* be done and results can be obtained. No one except French has attempted experimentation of this type before. It is quite possible that an independent group outside of the industry should be funded to produce an organized research effort to systematically determine specific and verifiable information and procedures for the design of seating, especially seating for the elderly.

Function of the Specific Seating Type

Observations made during the research of Koncelik, Ostrander, and Snyder (1972) reveal that probably no more than seven functional types of seating are currently used in the nursing home. Although there are variations and hybrids, these functional types include (1) the mobile geriatric chair, (2) the wheelchair, (3) stationary geriatric chairs, (4) lounge chairs, (5) side chairs, (6) dining chairs, and (7) occasional chairs or temporary seating.

The most critical seating problems are found in the design of the seating used by the nonambulatory patient-residents. This includes the mobile geriatric chair, the wheelchair, and the stationary geriatric chair. The first two types of seating are used throughout the day and are multifunctional. Durations of seated time and specific functions of these chairs have been discussed throughout this text. The third type of seating is more difficult to describe in terms of specific function according to observation data. The stationary geriatric chair is really a specialized furnishing that should be used for transfers from the bed of nonambulatory and highly disabled patient-residents. It is a method of having these patient-residents assume a seated position to relieve them of constant supine positions assumed in the bed, thus providing an alternative posture and possible prevention of decubitus ulcers. The chair should be designed to accommodate incontinence and restraint-support.

Unfortunately, as currently found in nursing homes, this chair is mistakenly cast as a lounge chair for ambulatory patient-residents. This is an inappropriate use of the chair. It is also an inappropriate specification for the *design* of this chair. Outside of the patient-resident room, transfers from the mobile geriatric chair and the wheelchair are infrequent, so that a stationary geriatric chair is not going to receive heavy use. It is possible that when a patient-resident who is nonambulatory needs his own stationary seating to perform some task or indulge in activities, the geriatric chair might be located outside of the patient-

FIGURE 68

Chairs with additional softening materials. Regardless of the design, purpose, or configuration, one of the most serious problems in providing adequate chair comfort is eliminating the abrasive feel of hardness that comes from inadequate spring base support. No matter how much softening material is added to the surface, the problem remains, especially because the elderly sit for such extended periods of time. (Photo: John Kelsey and Robert Steinbugler.)

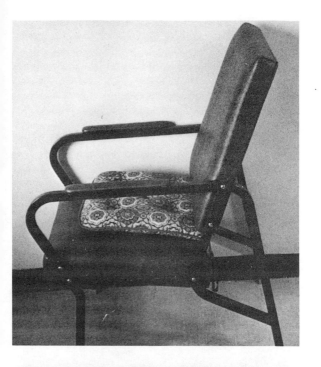

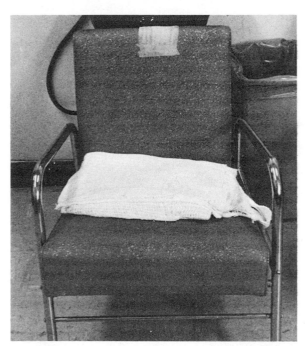

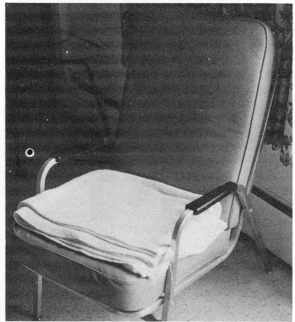

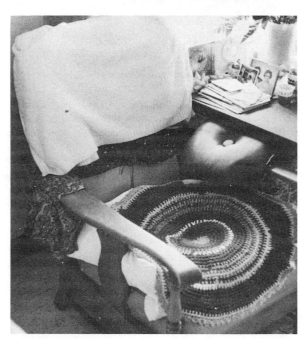

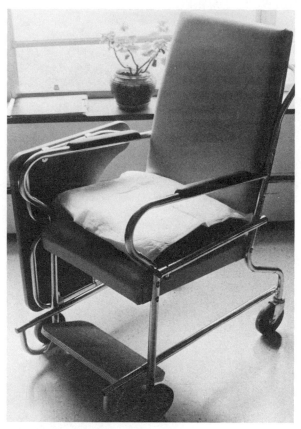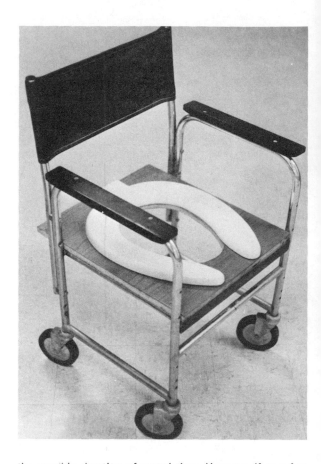

FIGURE 69

Intrainstitutional transportation seating. It has been shown quite frequently through observations that there are at least two types of mobile chairs needed in nursing homes, yet only one is designed for its intended purpose. The geriatric wheelchair or "restraint" chair is a mobile, staff-propelled, long-term seating device; note the incontinence pad, which suggests the possible duration of seated time. However, if transfers are going to be made, often lighter chairs are used because they are more maneuverable and easier to push, although their comfort is a matter of serious question. (Photo: John Kelsey and Robert Steinbugler.)

resident room. However, this implies more general usage will not be made of the chair, and it might become an obstruction that must be moved after use.

Lounge chairs and side chairs are designed for the ambulatory patient-resident. They should be located in places outside the patient-resident room as well as in the patient-resident room. It is important to remain flexible concerning the location of furnishings in any part of the facility. Some patient-residents are going to require stationary geriatric seating and sufficient space for a mobile geriatric chair. Others, who may be ambulatory, will need lounge chairs or may desire their own personal seating in their rooms.

The lounge chair should be designed to support the patient-resident while seated both awake and sleeping. It should be designed around the premise of continence and *not* incontinence. This means that lounge seating should be *fabric covered* or of breath-

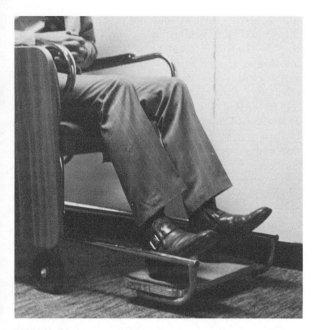

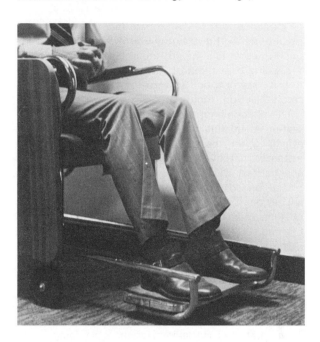

FIGURE 70

Foot-rest positions. As the feet are extended or swung from the knee, there is a need to keep them perpendicular to the line of the leg and not at an excessive obtuse angle. With the toes raised, the shin becomes less vulnerable to receiving blows from other wheelchair foot rests, especially under tables where the distance of penetration is difficult to judge. (Photo: John Kelsey and Robert Steinbugler.)

able vinyls for comfort for long durations. Armrests should extend beyond the leading edge of the seat platform so that the patient–resident can pull himself or herself from the chair after a protracted duration. The ends of the rest should offer an enlarged, upturned gripping surface so that an arthritic hand can easily form about the surface and purchase for grip. Legs should be sufficiently splayed to contact floor surfaces at four points outside the periphery of the seat platform. Cantilever designs for leg configurations are largely inappropriate and are frequently too springy.

All seating that is used for long durations should conform to similar, if not identical, deflection and spring–damping rate criteria. There is no necessity for any lounge chairs that employ foam only or foam and spring supports to deflect beyond 2 inches to provide an adequate cushioning. Excessive deflections in the chair will constrict the open angle of the torso and make egress from the chair more difficult.

Deflection into the seat platform has two aspects that should be noted. First is "initial feel." Initial feel refers to the sensation of relative softness or cushioning a chair provides at the moment of entrance deflection. The second aspect is "ride," or how the support cushioning feels over the entire duration period of the occupancy. A chair with extremely pleasant initial feel might have very poor ride, or vice versa. Therefore, the person selecting chairs should be aware that one sitting in a showroom will not provide all the information necessary to make a sound judgment.

Providing adequate "ride" in a chair, especially a chair meant for long seated durations, means providing a spring base in the seat platform. Without a spring base, there will be a fixed limit to deflection and "bottoming out" in the chair. This refers to the chair reaching a point where deflection stops completely. A lounge chair or long duration seat of any type should be provided with a spring base that will deflect to a predetermined limit, but will provide more deflection under greater load or shifting in the seat. Technically, the spring base should be so designed that its deflection is "asymptotic" to zero—or that it never reaches zero deflection (Figure 65).

The phenomenon of "bottoming" in long duration seating in nursing homes has curious and observable effects upon the people and the seating in some instances. Frequently, observers will note several applications of materials on seats. Pillows will be placed on foam pads, on the top of soft blankets, and so on. There is sometimes a buildup of materials on seats to make them "softer" over a longer period of time. Unfortunately, none of the applications of materials will resolve the problem, because after the initial feel characteristic has dissipated, the seat is still bottoming and continuing to exert pressure upon the posterior at the ischial tuberosities support points. This will provide a rubbing sensation that cannot be alleviated through soft materials on the top surface. These materials actually offer more damping in the seat mechanism and may even hasten the discomfort (see Figures 67 and 68).

A great deal of experimentation needs to be done to determine correct combinations of materials for seat platforms and seat back cushions. There is science, technology, and art in the design of these characteristics and resulting configurations. Although the approach must be systematic in order to develop verifiable results in the procedures and evaluations, there are too many variable aspects to consider this type of seating design anything but a subjective task. However, to further identify the nature of the task, the effort should be classified as attempts to provide *suspension* seating rather than *nonsuspension* seating. Nonsuspension seating for the nursing home would be the classification for functional seating, such as dining room or activity station seating.

One further note of importance regarding long duration seating. The seat platform and the seat back cushion should remain independent of one another. These two elements should not be tied together or developed as a single sling from top to leading edge of the seat platform. This type of development is appropriate for semisupine and fully

supine seating devices, but the erect seating posture should not be supported in a sling. The phenomenon that develops is referred to as "hammocking." When pressure is applied to either the seat platform or the seat back cushion, the other tightens. The resulting effect is a rocking back and forth in the seat from top to leading edge in compensation for the transfers of tension in the material. This provides very unsatisfactory seating, because there can be no shift of position in the seat that will provide continued or improved comfort.

Side chairs must be regarded in the same category as other long duration seating, since a suspension mechanism should be provided as the support device in the construction of the seat. However, the use of side chairs is less specific in nursing homes, and the durations of seated times are probably less than that for lounge chairs or mobile seating with all of their multifunctionality. Side chairs are often provided as a companion device to the bed to permit conversations between the bed occupant and the visitor. They may be found in lounges and entrance areas of the nursing home.

A chief consideration for the side chair is that it may be the appropriate device for the nongeriatric person. Sufficient seating must be provided throughout the facility for those who visit or volunteer their time as companions or assistants in the nursing home. The side chair, with its ease of movability (it should be light enough to move) and comfort seems the appropriate device for this function.

Dining chairs are the most critical functional chair type found in the nursing home. They must be regarded as having the one function for which they are designed. To expedite the dining function there must be adequate support in the lower back and lumbar region. As mentioned earlier, the elderly patient-resident will rely completely for support to the back on the seat back. Although the nongeriatric dining chair user may lean forward to compensate for the distance between the chair back and table edge, the elderly user will not.

Although the chair should have arms for entrance and egress, the arms should penetrate beneath the support apron of the table. As in other stationary furnishings, the dining chair should be four legged, and the points of contact with the floor should be in a square periphery outside the seat platform periphery (Figure 55).

Occasional seating is really a catchall for seating that does not suit the classifications, but more importantly includes seating which may be moved into a space temporarily for meetings or other functions. One important problem to be reconciled in this type of seating is the possibility for slippage on slick surfaces. Although this criterion applies to other forms of seating as well, the light chair with less spread to the legs for support will be more susceptible to sliding and possible toppling during the process of entrance and egress.

The typical folding chair may present problems in regard to these criteria. It is improbable that there is a great chance of specialized furnishings of this kind being developed for nursing homes. Other markets produce the largest proportion of sales. The designer and the administrator who must select furniture of this type must choose carefully to ensure that the types of chairs chosen will provide the necessary support to the user.

The criteria mentioned so far relate to the design of seating; but the same criteria relate just as strongly to the selection of seating and chairs in general as well. Whether it is the designer or the administrator or a selected staff member who is choosing seating for an institution, the criteria discussed should be used as a guide.

Simple tests can be devised when inspecting seating devices for purchase or just casually observing the seating utilized in a facility. First, the chair—if light enough—should be turned upside down so that the manufacturer can be noted and so that two important functional constructional details can be observed. First, the method of affixing the seat trim to the underside of the chair should be observed. Second, there should be some form of corner bracing or blocking to tie the sides of the chair together and stabilize the chair if it is of wooden construction. This construction detail will also stabilize the legs to some degree. Designs vary and materials vary, so there are a great number of adequate design techniques that enable the manufacturer to make a sturdy and stable chair. However, generally speaking, the overall finish and attention to detail will provide many clues to the quality of the product.

The bottoming characteristic can be easily tested for by plunging the clenched fist into the center of the seat cushion in a straight, steady, and increasingly forceful manner. If there is an abrupt stopping where no deflection is rendered in spite of increase of force, it is probable that the seat bottoms. Obviously, when the chair is upside down and a rigid platform is observed, the chair will most definitely bottom.

When making selections for the patient-residents in the nursing home, there are chairs that should be avoided. Any couch over two seated positions in length is unsuitable for patient-resident occupancy. Once there are three positions designed into the configuration of a couch, there is no way that the patient-resident will be able to extract himself or herself from the seated position. Even at the outer positions, there is insufficient graspable condition presented with only one chair arm usable for egress. As a general rule, avoid putting couches in patient-resident accessible spaces.

Avoid ganged seating. First, this places everyone at a side-by-side position, which prevents conversation. Second, ganged seating is often prone to interaction as people enter and egress. Every time someone enters or leaves the seating device, everyone else who is seated feels it. Some ganged seating is so interactive that when one person leaves, everyone leaves.

Anyone selecting seating should be very careful about seating with a high degree of spring in the legs, supports, or through the base. There are rockers available built with metal springs as leg members. These chairs present an extremely unstable entrance-egress condition.

Generally, all rules of common sense apply in the selection of chairs and seating devices. It would be very desirable to see far fewer static seating devices purchased for nursing homes and those that are purchased bought with greater care.

Research and Development of New Seating

In view of the lack of systematic methods for developing really good seating for nursing homes and the absence of uniform evaluation methods to determine the adequacy of any given seating development, there should be an intensive research and development effort to develop this technology. It is improbable that, like the automotive industry, where the self-interest and capital exist, the institutional furnishings industry will be an effective instrument to develop such information.

Aside from the techniques to develop and evaluate seating, there is a pressing need to explore developments of new seating types. Some possible directions are suggested in this text; however, there are more specific directions that could prove fruitful. The development of a mobile geriatric chair and wheelchair that are more visually and structurally alike is one example. The inferences of what the difference between the two chairs means to the population are significant in that some patient–residents are identified as "sicker" than others by virtue of the chair they occupy. A basic frame and suspension seat, which could be applied to both types of seating, could be interchangeable with the external mobile chassis that provides either self-powered actuation or assisted mobility. Another possibility is a motorized wheelchair that could be given to nonambulatory but psychologically unimpaired patient–residents to promote greater mobility throughout the facility.

In view of the extended durations of seated time, it is certainly feasible and possibly very desirable to design seating which can vary or adjust in angularity so that there can be change of position. This might be very useful in avoiding decubitus ulcers and maintaining comfort over long periods of time.

Other possibilities include a more specialized stationary geriatric chair, including exploration of different configurations of materials and contour in view of the cleaning problem. Lounge chairs could be far more extensively developed to support and provide comfort as well as vary or adjust.

These are but a few of the possible design developments that should be explored. The state of the art in seating design for nursing homes can be described as stagnant. The principles, seating types, and assumed human factors and needs have remained almost absolutely stable for at least 30 years. Yet most designers and engineers who work in other fields—especially in the vehicular seating field—are aware of technologies and design methods that go far beyond the state of the art in the institutional furnishings field.

Applications of New Technology

The distance between the seating industry in other areas and that of the institutional furnishings industry in the application of design techniques and evaluation criterion is equalled by the lack of application of new materials and production techniques in the furnishings industry. There have been many new developments in spring media for spring bases for seating over the past decade and more; but little of what has been done is yet applied to the nursing home furnishings. Rubber spring platforms, full foam platforms in molded buckets, and webbing used as spring media are some of the new material developments. Restraint might be provided through belts on retraction reels, just as in automotive seating. Silicone gel cushions are already available on the market today for use as cushions to relieve the incidence of decubitus ulcers. The precise technology used to develop this product is not explored sufficiently at this point and may hold great promise as a device employed directly as a seat cushion.

An infinite variety of possible design solutions hold great promise for better seating for patient–residents in nursing homes. Because of the stagnation of the technology in this area and the lack of design development over the years, almost too much really needs to be done and should be done. It remains to be seen whether or not the appropriate energy will be expended to upgrade the seating now being used.

Problems in Manufacturing and Distribution

Some of the problems in developing new seating through the existing network of the industry concerned with this product area have been touched upon. There is a large abundance of undercapitalized manufacturers operating in the field; very few have design staffs or employ design at any point; there is little effort applied to a coordinated attempt to develop standards. Manufacturers in the institutional furnishings field do not distribute over large sections of the country for the most part. There is very little coordination of a full-force sales approach and, excepting the largest manufacturers in the field, no advertising outside the distribution of brochures. To a great degree, the line of institutional furnishings offered outside of chair production is basically a line of hospital furnishings either translated or stepped down in the number of offerings. There is little interest among manufacturers in research and development of new products because there must be an absolute guarantee that the product will sell in sufficient quantities to justify time spent in development. Basically, the sales effort in this field is a door-to-door approach. Conferences and conventions offer the only organized, high-impact sales effort in this field.

The problems that affect the manufacturing of equipment in this field affect the entire health care field. The production of specialized goods for nursing homes can be projected as just part of a larger problem—no unified or agglomerated market. The changes necessary to upgrade any line of products become possible as the number of products in production rises. There is a tremendous contrast between the manufacturing of geriatric chairs, which may be done on a batch basis and practically all hand fabricated in lots of a few hundred, and General Motors production of over 4 million bucket seats.

In essence, the manufacturer is forced to stay close to the market place and not deviate from the accepted norm of products almost every designer and administrator accepts. This presents grave problems if the equipment used in nursing homes is ever to improve. There must be an external force, external to manufacturing, that makes possible the necessary research and development.

One clear prospect is the voluntary combination of nursing homes in an association to form an agglomerated market. If the members of the nursing home field, the administrators, staffs, and design consultants, realize that they have common needs which can only be satisfied by combining efforts, an agglomerated market might be formed. In a very short time, separate entities that order in lots of hundreds or less become associations ordering in lots of thousands.

The pattern of buying that this effort would parallel is that of every other industry where mass production exists. In the mobile home industry, for example, quantity buying has enabled manufacturers to obtain reduced prices on each individual item; they are also able to demand products that meet their specifications.

Another example of change in product design in the health care area is the interesting case of the British Ministry of Health, which sponsored a research and development program under the auspices of a research unit at the Royal College of Art to develop new beds. In this instance a full research program was launched in which the needs of hospitals all over the British Isles were ascertained and computerized. After an intensive analysis of the collected information, a design program was launched, culminating in the limited production of 50 prototypes that were field tested. When the product had been thoroughly evaluated over a period of time, the ministry combined the requirements for beds of a large number of hospitals, let out the bed design for bids, selected a manufacturer, and provided an initial order of *7000 beds*!

Owing to the success of this first design program, the Ministry of Health has pushed forward in many other product areas, including the development of specialized products for the home that will enable children to care for their parents at home in spite of health problems including incontinence.

Obviously, there are controls that can be used in a socialized health care system which cannot be administered in a free market health care system. Also, the case study of this extraordinary example of development in the health care field of a socialized health care nation is not to be construed as an argument for that type of system in this country. However, this country is rapidly falling behind other countries that employ socialized health care and others that do not have a national health care system in the development of new products, as well as other aspects of health care. The nursing home field in the United States must find its own answer in permitting or fostering new development or remain in the same position it has occupied for the past 30 years or more.

FURNISHINGS

Aside from seating and beds, furnishings that should receive special attention are tables, open storage units, and case goods (dressers, bureaus, etc.). It is safe to say that these items receive the least amount of specialization for nursing home use; yet, definite and specific requirements should be met to ensure the usefulness and safety of these items in the nursing home setting.

Tables have been discussed in other sections of the text, especially the requirement that all tables selected be of the 30-inch-height variety and not low coffee tables, which are essentially functionless and obstructive to use of space in the nursing home. In addition, the texture of the table surface should afford purchase for dry hands when gripping is necessary for rising or in sitting. The top surface should not be white or too light so that there is excessive reflection of light or glare. Glassware, papers, and other items will be lost on a pure white surface, especially in high-glare situations.

The edge of the table should be rolled, not cut square in cross section or sharp edged. There should be sufficient cross section for gripping, and the blunted edge would reduce the prospect of injury during a fall.

The legs of the table should be clearly marked at the lower ends to promote visibility, so that the older person has a sense of where the leg is when he or she turns to move away from the table or can see it while approaching to be seated.

The apron of the table, or support frame, should be designed to permit the penetration of the standard dining room chair with arms (which may or may not be a matching set), the mobile geriatric chair used in the facility, and the wheelchair. This is an extremely broad range to accommodate with one fixed table design. It is possible that two tables must be selected for a given facility with slight variations in height.

The number of persons at a given table is discussed in the section on the dining room and is part of the planning and design of this space. Conversational groupings should be limited in number to be effective. The needs that any given facility present may vary, and fixing the number per table or selecting a table that can only accommodate four might not always be the most desirable.

One of the most important problems to be reckoned with in the dining room is the segregation of patients according to capability. It is desirable to have the patients in wheelchairs and in geriatric chairs mixed with the ambulatory as much as possible. Yet, there is the problem of decrements in ability to feed independently. Administrators report on occasion that they feel strongly that the capable elderly should be allowed to dine with others who are as capable as they are. This is perhaps the only degree of permissible segregation in the nursing home. However, extreme care must be exercised in the determination of just who among the total population should be screened out for assisted feeding. Dysfunction of the lower extremities does not necessarily mean that there is concurrent mental or other physiological difficulty which would impair the ability to dine independently.

The open storage (display) and case goods that should receive the primary attention from designers are those items found in the patient–resident room. Other storage and case goods outside of this space would be supervised by staff, and their use would be limited and scrutinized. Thus, the first consideration is the safety of those patient–residents who are using furnishings in the privacy of their rooms and are not being supervised.

There should be a minimum radius determined for the edges of all hard surfaces and protrusions that present possible injury-producing projections in the tight spaces of the patient–resident room. This would not be very difficult. Automotive safety specifications call for a minimum radius on all knobs, dials, edges of dashboard surfaces, and the like. The velocity of impact could be calculated for the falling body and measurements of impact force deduced, especially at the head. A minimum radius could be determined from the data by selecting an impact force less than that capable of causing severe injury (fracture of the skull) to the head. The more a corner is rounded off, the broader the impact area and the more dispersed the force of the blow. It would be very desirable to begin employing a radius on edges and corners of institutional storage units and case goods as a precaution even now, without a formal specification.

Another important safety consideration is that these furnishings are going to be used as supports while walking or braces while performing some task in the room. No storage unit or case goods unit should be selected that is not sufficiently stable to act as a brace or support. Storage units that are modular and utilize vertical pole or column members will be very susceptible to this kind of use. Their mounting points must be very stable, and single pole units should be avoided completely. The shelving on the units should also be stable enough to support use as a grab rail. Many storage systems utilize horizontal members that simply rest upon other support members. These will shift when grasped and should not be specified for use in nursing home settings.

Goldsmith's *Designing for the Disabled* (1967) is perhaps the most authoritative text on environments for handicapped people, especially those confined to wheelchairs. Goldsmith makes the astute observation that the conditions or criteria of design of a room for a wheelchair-bound person and an ambulatory person are sufficiently different that the designs should vary. There is an unfortunate trend toward compromise of these criteria, attempts in many institutional designs and residential designs to compromise the dimensional criteria to arrive at one set of dimensions for both groups of users. These compromises usually mean that neither group is served well. This is not a viable approach in the setup of patient–residents' rooms for the nursing home. This philosophy especially applies to the selection and design of surface heights, limits of penetration, placement of drawers, and other aspects of storage and case goods design (Figure 21).

It is entirely possible that the storage units and case goods units in a patient–resident room could and should be variable: modular units could be suspended from a wall-mounted or free-standing rack system, allowing two basic variations in height setup depending on the ambulatory status of the patient–resident who will occupy the space. There are systems available on the market today that allow for variations in height of kitchen cabinetry depending on the height of the user. This equipment is sometimes provided for apartment dwellings and can be adjusted prior to entry for a new tenant. The consumer market is very likely to see many more variable units in production in the coming years. However, it is in the institutional setting that the greatest applicability for these devices, and the greatest need, exists.

All too frequently, general-purpose work surfaces, such as cosmetics or grooming areas, will have a height determined by a storage unit below with a standard arrangement of drawers. This type of case goods is totally inappropriate for the wheelchair-bound user. There should be sufficient space beneath the surface for the penetration of the legs of the user. This could mean that only one shallow drawer beneath a surface is permissible to allow for the penetration needed to affect proper utilization of the device. Full-length drawer units should have an 8-inch-high by 3-inch-deep kick space at the base of the item to allow for penetration of the foot rests of the wheelchair, and to prevent scrubbing and marring of wood surfaces or other surfaces that would be contacted by the wheelchair during movement (Figures 69 and 70).

Mirrors which may be mounted to the rear of cosmetic stands should be flush to the backsplash of a surface no more than 30 inches high. Mirrors should be canted forward at the top edge to expedite use by the wheelchair-bound person. The cant should be no more than 5 degrees so that the visual feedback is primarily of the face and not the top of the head and lap or counter surface.

Storage systems that employ shelving beyond the reach of the wheelchair-bound patient–resident in a room occupied by a person of this ambulatory status will not be used as a primary storage area, although items not in use may be placed out of reach by others acting for the wheelchair-bound patient–resident. Drawers that are effectively blocked by the knees and side chair structure will also fall out of use unless they can be approached and opened from the side. Thus, an internal track system inside case goods must allow for side forces and prevent racking when these side forces are applied. Filing cabinets utilize such a mechanical system. A force exerted on any corner to open the drawer will not cause racking.

This use also requires that there not be center drawer pulls used on institutional case goods. There

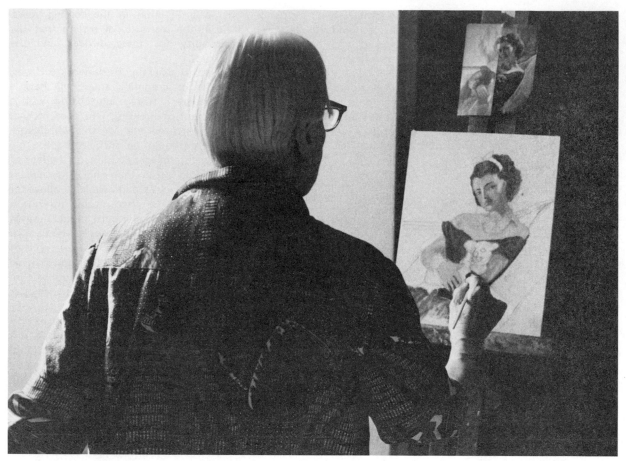

FIGURE 71

The range of activities in the control of patient–residents within their own space must be extended. "Control" over space implies that the use of space is the prerogative of the patient-resident. Activities are of *their* choosing—just as the various physical amenities (light, heat, and so on) are under their control. (Photo: David O. Watkins.)

are several options: a full lip extending the length of the drawer, large graspable drawer pulls on two sides of the drawers, and combinations of handles and pulls, which also might present interesting formal as well as human factors solutions.

BED AND BEDDING

H. M. Parsons has written extensively on the bedroom. The fundamental point he develops (1972)

quite clearly is the idea that the bed is a surface upon which, around which, and because of which many different behaviors and needs occur. There are sleeping behaviors, resting behaviors, sexual activities, and cleaning and changing activities, all of which must be accounted for in the development of the bed for particular users and environments.

A great proportion of the daily activity of the patient-resident begins and ends at the bed. To consider the bed as simply a place to sleep is to deny the many other functions Parsons has noted as relevant to bed design.

The nursing home bed can be seen as a control center of the room. From the bed, the bulk of the space and objects in that space should be visible or within view with little difficulty of movement. The controls for light, sound and music, television, communications, temperature and air control, natural light screening, nurse call and communications, and other signaling devices should be organized as a surround within reach of the bed. The control surfaces should be shape-coded for recognition by sight-impaired persons and color-coded for easy differentiation for those with lesser problems of sight. In addition, there should be an orientation session with staff members for the new patient–resident regarding the control devices and practice sessions to establish their proper use (see Figures 15, 17, and 18).

This "bed surround" should also include storage units for reading materials, nonperishable foods if permissible, glasses, hearing aids, illuminated magnifiers, writing materials, and other paraphernalia that might be used while the patient–resident is resting in a semisupine position (Figures 15 and 17).

In addition to storage and controls area, the bed surround should be equipped with a retractable and adjustable writing or work surface, which might also double as an eating surface for the bedridden.

Several possibilities are feasible technically for the design of such a complex. The "surround" itself might be a detachable unit of free-standing members or units to which a bed is connected. The bed itself might either pull away manually for changing or might be motorized and driven outward and away for cleaning and changing from the surround itself (see Figure 17). Mechanisms currently exist and are used in a vast array of products that could be incorporated in the design of such a product. Any discussion of costs must be balanced against the incorporation of many of the same devices in separate units or in the architecture—making the design inflexible and out of reach.

For the most part, modern nursing homes have control devices incorporated in wall panels in back of the bed. There are nurses' call buttons on long wires or tubes. These devices are often unreachable or usu-

ally become entangled in the bedding of the room occupant. Essentially, this proposal is an attempt to organize items in a more convenient manner and to provide the identifiability necessary to ensure their appropriate use.

The bed surface itself should be larger (longer and wider) than is currently the standard found in nursing homes. Greater attention should be given to the width and length of the bed, but a reasonable estimate of the increase is that the bed should be one and a half times the current width and possibly 7 feet in length.

There are two basic reasons for providing greater width in the bed surface. First, as Parsons has stated (1972), the wider the bed, the more potential there is for different positions and movement of the body during sleep and resting. Second, the healthier patient–resident with a living spouse or a love partner should have the opportunity and the privacy for lovemaking.

Lengthening the bed surface will be necessary as an accommodation to a population that will increase in height quite rapidly over the next two decades, as well as to provide a longer platform for movement and resting positions.

Additional research and development studies should be undertaken to determine many functional aspects of the bed used in nursing homes. The number of positions the bed may assume should not be an outgrowth of the physiological determinants of the hospital bed. The depth of deflection, spring rate, suspension members, and support given to the body should be studied. In addition, there might be an effort launched to determine the best combination of materials and/or mechanical devices, such as forced air through the surface of the bed, to prevent or to heal decubitus ulcers.

There is also the extreme situation where life support equipment or testing equipment must be brought into the room and positioned near the bed. The equipment that must be accommodated for these periods are the suction machine, which extracts fluids from the trachea, the oxygen tank and canopy or mask equipment, and the electrocardiograph machine. It would be rare to have all in use at the same time, but it is recommended that a location be predetermined at the bedside—perhaps as part of the surround—where

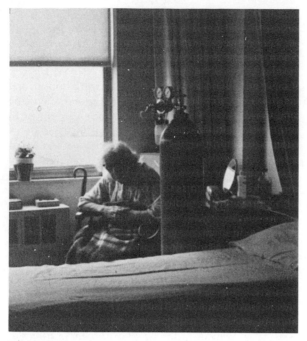

FIGURE 72
Spatial interference from a dangerous object. (Photo: David
O. Watkins.)

each of these items or equipment can be accommodated and used without interfering with the other.
Without this consideration, dangerous interference
to room circulation can result (Figure 72).

Another consideration is that the visual impact of
these devices is very strong and conveys advanced
illness or impending death. There should not be such
hesitancy on the part of friends, cohorts, and relatives
when this equipment is near at hand that conversations are cut off or fear is conveyed to the patient–
resident.

The oxygen tank presents a design problem in itself.
There is no difference between the tank used in
nursing homes and those used on construction sites
for oxyacetylene welding. The same imposing, rusted,
and crude device is wheeled into a patient–resident's
room as that hauled up a steel structure to weld beams
and columns. It is dangerous in that, when knocked
over, the top might detach and suddenly a jet-pro-

pelled bomb is loose inside a room. Codes require
that oxygen tanks be chained to the wall to prevent
their being tipped over or moved about. Unfortunately,
because of the use made of tanks and the necessity
of constant resupply, chaining is frequently not done.
The bottle is tall and narrow and susceptible to tipping. It is also very heavy, and if any difficulty occurs
with a friend or relative in the room, they may be
unable to quickly react and right the bottle.

The best container for compressed gasses is a completely spherical container. The volume of a container
of this sort, comparable to that of the standard oxygen
tank would subsume a shape lower in profile and far
less susceptible to tipping. The diameter, of course,
increases, but this is a price worth paying to achieve
greater safety and less conspicuousness in design.

The bedding used in nursing homes, as well as the
garments worn in bed, need study and the application of techniques of fastening and wrapping that
might expedite self-clothing and self-help in making
the bed. Bedding per se should be attractive and
personal if at all possible, especially the top dressing
of the bed.

One neglected area is the space directly overhead
the patient-resident when occupying the bed. When
consideration is given to the bedridden and the
blankness of this aspect of the environment, it is
plain that some attention could be given to treating
the ceiling or providing visual or auditory communications or entertainment for this group of
patient-residents. Like the mobile geriatric chair,
the bed and its immediate surroundings becomes an
environment, the only environment for some members of the nursing home population. There is no
reason why this environment cannot be enriched and
stimulating for those who otherwise pass hours unoccupied.

It is possible that a return to the canopy or four
poster in a new variation might be an answer to the
problem becoming the environment for the bedridden. Certainly it is possible to design a structure
that could support a variety of visual, auditory, and
tactile stimuli for the enjoyment of someone who is
faced with constant confinement to the bed. When
there is an emergency, this structure could be en-
shrouded easily for the use of environmental controls

such as oxygen, intravenous therapies, and other medical equipment.

Perhaps the central point to be remembered regarding the furnishings mentioned as part of the patient–resident's microenvironment is that they are the more important "prostheses" in the whole physical environment. They act as physical and psychological supports. They must provide control, comfort, stimulation, and a sense of positiveness about the overall environment.

REFERENCES

French, Michael. "Posture Changes in Relationship to Variations in Seat Trim Among the Elderly Infirm." In *First Community Village Research Report*, Joseph A. Koncelik (ed.). Unpublished Manuscript. Columbus, O.: Department of Industrial Design, Ohio State University, 1975.

Goldsmith, Selwyn. *Designing for the Disabled.* London: Royal Institute of British Architects, 1967.

Kira, Alexander. *The Bathroom: Criteria for Design.* Ithaca, N.Y.: Cornell University Center for Housing and Environmental Studies, 1966.

Koncelik, Joseph A., Edward Ostrander, and Lorraine H. Snyder. *The Relationship of the Physical Environment in 6 Extended Care Facilities to the Behavior of Their Resident Aging People.* Research Report No. 103. Ithaca, N.Y.: Department of Design and Environmental Analysis, College of Human Ecology, Cornell University, 1972.

Laging, Barbara. "Who Are the Elderly." *The Designer*, 16, no. 180 (1972), p. 4.

Parsons, Henry M. "The Bedroom." *Human Factors*, 15, no. 5 (1972), pp. 421–450.

President's Committee on Employment of the Handicapped. Recommendations of the Subcommittee on Barrier Free Design, Pamphlet ANSI Standard 117.1, *Making Buildings Accessible and Usable by the Physically Handicapped.* Washington, D.C.: Superintendent of Documents. 1971.

Snyder, Lorraine H. "A Case in Point: The Geriatric Wheel Chair." *The Human Ecology Forum*, 3, no. 2 (1972), pp. 7–9.

——, Edward Ostrander, J. A. Koncelik. *The New Nursing Home: Conference Proceedings.* Ithaca, N.Y.: College of Human Ecology, Cornell University, June 1973, pp. 37–47.

U.S. Department of Health, Education and Welfare, Public Health Service. *Weight, Height, and Selected Body Dimensions of Adults: United States—1960–1962*, series 11, no. 8. Washington, D.C.: National Center for Health Statistics, 1965.

RECOMMENDATIONS FOR ARCHITECTURAL DETAILS

Architectural details that are of importance in the context of openness in nursing home design are those products, building components, and devices with which the patient–resident has contact or directly that affect his or her existence in some way. There is a hazy area of product design and building fixture design, which does affect the patient–resident to some degree, but with which he is in potentially limited contact, that requires special attention in and of itself. This area includes such items as food service products, delivery carts, and microwave ovens. Heating, ventilation, and cooling systems and the general mechanical core also fit in this area; the patient–resident exerts some control over them or is affected by them, but the products require a greater degree of investigation and recommendations that can be afforded in this text.

No part of this text has been concerned nor can it be concerned with the total service of the nursing home. The design of kitchens, materials handling areas, staff meeting rooms, administration offices, and other aspects of the system which are removed from the patient–resident cannot be given the attention they merit.

Under the heading of architectural details are 13 items that must be discussed and for which recommendations must be developed. These items have an important impact upon the user, either because the user must perform some task manipulating them or they influence the user's daily life. These items are the following:

1. Electrical outlets and switches.
2. Lighting devices and controls.
3. Telephones.
4. Electrical product controls.
5. Communications devices and bulletin boards.
6. Doors and door handles.
7. Fixed ambulatory aids, handrails, and supports.
8. Safety devices and fire doors.
9. Wall finishes and surfaces.
10. Materials for decor and identification.
11. Color and color coding.
12. Windows and glazed surfaces.
13. Sound attenuating devices.

ELECTRICAL OUTLETS AND SWITCHES

Generally, the outlet mounted at a height of 16 to 20 inches above the floor will be more satisfactory than those mounted at standard architectural heights.

This dimension should be measured from the baseplate of the outlet to the floor surface. It should be possible for the wheelchair user to reach to the bottom of most sockets in the two-outlet plate and either insert or retract a plug. The selection of the plug type is just as important as the outlet itself. There should be a graspable surface, with possibly a hook or loop for ease of grasp. The wire should either project downward directly from the plug or to the side. One serious problem with high mounted outlets is that they allow the projection of wires perpendicular to the wall surface. This presents a definite hazard to both the ambulatory patient–resident and the wheelchair user. The outlet should contrast in value of color with the plug so that they can be easily seen and matched (Figure 73).

Wall-mounted switches should be lower than the standard placement found in most buildings. Switches in areas where no grab rails are found should be mounted at 32 inches off the floor to the baseplate of the switch in order to expedite use by the wheelchair-bound user. It would be of considerable benefit to use switches that could be palmed as well as moved with the finger. The switch itself should be illuminated and there should be provision on the baseplate for graphic identification of the switch controls.

LIGHTING DEVICES AND LIGHT SWITCHES

Light switches and the switches that are used to operate outlets are usually identical to each other, if not wired in the same baseplate. There should be some differentiation between the two types of switches either in terms of shape or color—perhaps graphically marked differently. Even in modern residential construction, occupants are forced to hunt and peck to find the proper switch for the light they want to turn on. Again, as with outlet switches, the switch should be illuminated and operable with the palm of the hand and not just fingers. There should also be a positive response or feedback in the switch signaling actuation (Figure 73).

Room and corridor lighting have been discussed in earlier sections of the text. However, it is worth reinforcing the point that single incandescent sources,

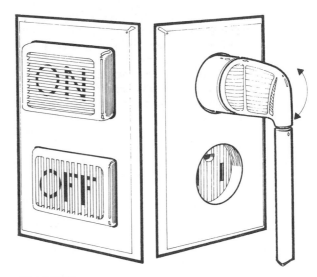

FIGURE 73

Switches and plugs. It is very important that these control elements be designed by manufacturers and chosen by architects with the human factors of the infirm elderly in mind. There is a loss of prehension and grasp strength associated with arthritis. The switch should be designed so that it can be actuated by the palm or the arm. The plug should be increased in surface area over current plugs on the market for sufficient grasping surface. The socket should have a recessed receiver so that the plug will virtually locate itself. The plug head should swivel so that the prongs do not twist depending on the direction of the cord.

whether or not there is one or more bulbs in the source, are poor design selections, although possibly the cheapest initial investment for a nursing home. Typically, a single source of this type is located in the center or near center of the space and is the only light used as general illumination. Space is poorly defined by a center light source. Corners, areas of the wall, and critical furnishings fall into shadow. The shadows formed by the light radiate in strong patterns out from the center of the room. Light falling on the face of a person moving through the space changes from a partial-subdued illumination to a strong contrasting light near the center of the room directly under or near the light. Obviously, floor lamps, reading lamps, and other general lighting over mirrors and in other locations change this effect and balance out the total illumination to some degree. This does require, however, that several lights be turned on, and most of them will be independently controlled. This would be impossible for the bedridden patient–resident; control would be out of his or her hands unless all controls were near the bed (Figure 15).

Within the "bed surround" there should be control(s) for the majority of the illumination in the space, including a dimmer switch to change the quantity of illumination. It is preferable that either valance or peripheral lighting schemes be used to effect a more uniform background for general lighting in the patient–resident room, dining spaces, lounge bays, and other areas. Lighting at the periphery of the space will define the walls and prevent harsh radiating shadows. People moving through space will retain a constant, though subdued, quantity and quality of illumination. Furnishings, generally located at the periphery of spaces, will be top lighted, with their surfaces readable and contents illuminated and visible (Figure 15).

There should be a light source mounted in the "bed surround" for reading and activities that might take place in bed. This source should be a balanced incandescent and fluorescent light source. The source should move freely but remain in position and not drift while an activity is in progress. Again, the switch should be readable and operable with the palm. The organization of elements and number of elements to be organized possibly means that the switch—as with all switches in the surround—should be shape- or texture coded.

So many different lighting products are available with so many differing characteristics that it is impossible to narrow down even a small group to recommend. However, the qualitative nature of the lighting systems is clear: there should be a warm rosy cast given to the skin by the light sources. Unfortunately, the cheapest fluorescents are frequently chosen for most institutional installations. These sources give off a blue-green cast to the environment. First, this emphasizes the worst characteristics of flesh tones and, second, the blue-green tones are the most difficult to perceive by the client population.

Specifications have been published that call for three times the quantity of illumination for environments for the elderly than in general settings. Yet observations show that this specification cannot be strictly adhered to nor is it adhered to in the large majority of facilities. A hard and fast specification of this kind is improper, because measurements can only be rendered directly under or around the light source. While one small area might have the properly specified quantity of light, the largest proportion of the area is not receiving that quantity.

There should be far more experimentation with lighting systems and schemes prior to construction. Scale models of spaces and lighting systems can often be very effective in giving a general and reasonably accurate picture of what a given lighting scheme will do to a space—and to its occupants and furnishings.

TELEPHONES

At least one public pay phone should be located in the corridor of every wing in the nursing home. The phone should be located on a wall at desk height (30 inches to the base from the floor) so that a wheelchair patient–resident can maneuver close to the phone and read the dial while dialing.

The dial should either be illuminated or have white letters and numerals on a black background. It would be preferrable to have a touch phone with audible tones actuated when the buttons are pushed. However, the dimensions of the buttons currently furnished on the standard AT&T telephone model with touch dial push buttons are too small, and the numerals and letters are too small for effective reading by sight-impaired persons. There is little chance of rectifying this problem until Bell Telephone decides to redesign current models.

The desirability of phones in every patient–resident room is questionable. However, an optional unit might be installed in the bed surround or a facia plate left in its absence. The phone is a part of life in the twentieth century, and its removal from the presence of an elderly person is one more indication of a loss of control and environmental inaccessibility.

ELECTRICAL PRODUCT CONTROLS

Attention has recently been given to the design of controls on the faceplates of modern electrical products with the idea in mind that a large number of consumers in the marketplace are "manipulatively handicapped." The ARMCO Steel Corporation sponsored a series of student projects in 1973–1974, which received a great deal of interest and attention (ARMCO Steel, 1974). The controls on television sets, radios, clocks, ranges, ovens, and the like, are all designed without consideration for literally millions of people who must use them daily and constitute a sizable segment of the market. The changes that need to be made are almost unbelievably simple, but they require recognition of the problem in the first place. The solutions applicable to that marketplace are also applicable for use in the nursing home and other specialized living units for the elderly. Knobs can be enlarged, different mechanisms employed (sliding bar controls), and graphics devised that would better communicate the proper use of the product (Figure 74).

COMMUNICATIONS DEVICES AND BULLETIN BOARDS

Very little is presently done inside the nursing home to inform patient–residents about events, lectures, parties, and other occurrences on an informal basis. Newsletters are prepared and announcements are made to groups, but providing some means of intrafacility communications is rare. Bulletin boards are usually considered sloppy and undesirable in facilities. They must be policed and old or improper notices taken down. Much of what ordinarily goes up on a bulletin board is written in a typeface so small as to be illegible by the majority of the population.

Tackboards or bulletin boards should be provided in spite of the problems they present in the facility. It could be possible for patient–residents to control monitoring of the boards and posting of notices. Large-type typewriters might be purchased and used by patient residents with typing skills who could run off notices and solicit internal communications.

Sharing and offering help are important compo-

nents of a total rehabilitation program. Whatever means, bulletin boards included, are used to foster these qualities among the patient–residents, the benefits to everyone, especially the staff, could be manifold.

Another communicative device rarely if ever used in institutional settings is the running of audiovisual equipment using patient–residents' materials as sources. Slide projectors could be located in key spots (lounge bays, dining rooms, etc.) where there could be guided accessibility and assistance. Slide projection equipment could be left running automatically, as in many exhibits, with travel slides, family albums, professional work, and art work, all used as a stimulus and entertainment media. Films and tape recordings could also be shared in much the same way.

Nursing homes are neglecting an aspect of almost every human being's life today by not taking advantage of the massive resource of audiovisual material most people have in their possession. Patient–residents could be encouraged to bring forth this material if the staff would start off showings from their own collections. Families and friends might be notified that such programming is going on, and they might bring forth additional material.

DOORS AND DOOR HANDLES

Life can be likened to constant passage through various types of portals. Indeed, doors play an important part in everyone's daily living. As with every other aspect of the physical environment of the nursing home, the door and door handle deserve great consideration because they are a chief barrier or facilitator in the lives of nursing home occupants.

The degree of ease with which a door can be opened or shut is inversely related to the increase in width. In the nursing home, doors are the widest of any used in institutional settings. Wheelchairs must pass through doorways; hoyer lifts and other devices must be transported from one space to another; and some patient–residents must be carried through doorways in times of emergency. Doors in nursing homes vary from just under 40 inches to over 48 inches. Occa-

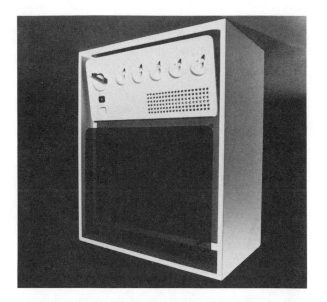

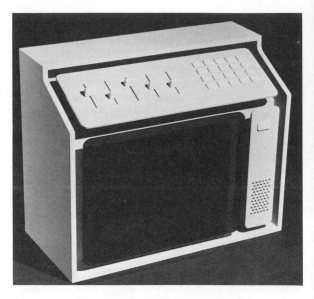

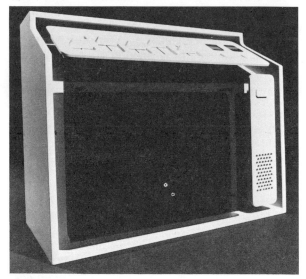

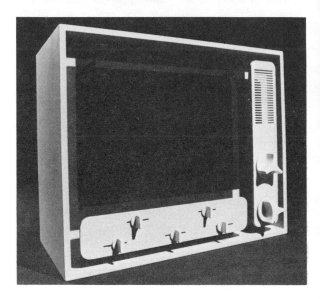

FIGURE 74

Variations on controls for products. The television sets shown were jointly designed by Ohio State University students James Besst, Michael French, John Samson, and Joseph Weidinger. As with the project on the design of a door latch, the focus was on making the device more ac-cessible for everyone by designing to the requirements of "special" users such as the handicapped. Products fol-lowing these user requirements would be additionally suitable for the inform elderly populations who reside in nursing homes. (Photo: Courtesy of ARMCO Steel Corporation.)

sionally, two-part doors are used; a standard-width door is combined with a flipper to provide even greater access into a space.

As the doors increase in size, so they increase in mass. The inertia a door of 48-inches width can build up when swung is considerable. Another added constraint is that the doors must be fire-rated and hung in a fire-rated "buck" or structural support mounted in the wall.

Because there are hinging systems that essentially eliminate resistance when an initial force is applied to open the door, there is little problem exhibited in getting doors to open. The first real problem is that a freely swinging fire-rated door can easily knock down an unseen person on the other side. Nurses and aids are often backing into a room carrying food trays or pulling carts. They are blind to any movement on the other side of a door, and thus a hazardous condition could arise.

One possible solution is the application of a door chime that must be rung prior to entry. This device would not only prevent accidents to some degree; it would reestablish a degree of privacy and control for the patient–resident. Visitors would need to be acknowledged prior to entry. For those who are hard of hearing, a light mounted in the room or at the bed surround might be employed to signal entry.

Doors in nursing homes are usually left open or even braced or fixed in the open position. Privacy is all but destroyed in these situations, and it is not necessary that every door to patient–resident rooms be constantly open. Obviously, where there are very ill patient–residents in bed who need the constant surveillance of staff, doors should be open to expedite watchfulness and entry.

Door surfaces need much more attention in the area of prevention of marring and abrasion. One unnoticed problem in virtually all nursing homes is the degree to which wheelchairs and other ambulatory aids hit the surface of doors, either upon entry and passage through the door or while the wheelchair user is passing down the hall using the handrail to pull the chair forward. In the latter case, where the handrail ends—at doorways—the wheelchair swings inward and hits the wall or door surface. Every door in a nursing home should be equipped with a buffer

plate or pad at the lower end to prevent marring from chair contact. This buffer plate should be continued down the hallway as well and at corners of the entryways in a vertical line where chipping will occur (Figure 32).

In addition, the hubs of wheelchairs and the leading edge of the footpads should be either coated with a plastic or taped to reduce marring wherever the wheelchair moves in the physical environment.

Door handles and locksets are a very important area for development for institutional use. It is important that a door handle provide sufficient surface and gripping area for the patient–resident to exert force either with the hand or with the lower arm. Thus, the standard knob is not the most desirable choice. Round, smooth surfaces are difficult to grip and actuate in a turning motion. A bar level device mounted to a standard latching mechanism is much more desirable. The surface of the door handle should be either round or ovaloid in cross section with no sharp edges. There are fixed door grips in use made from either pressed or molded steel stock with sharp edges. These are not only dangerous to the patient–residents in wheelchairs who contact the knob occasionally when entering or leaving a space; staff who open doors with hips also bruise themselves on latches and grips of this design (Figure 75).

Locksets and key inserts are often separated from the door latch mechanism. In either case, one important problem is the visualization of where the lock is and where or how to insert the key. Keys too are difficult to grip and actuate in the lock. Frequently, very precise locks jam and it is easy to twist off the shank of a key in a lock (Figures 75 and 76).

The shape of the lock insert should dish inward to direct the key toward the center and the insert. Flat smooth surfaces cause the key to skitter off and prevent easy tactile location of the insert. The insert area could be illuminated or at least treated in a bright color for ease of location.

The key itself should have a longer shank than normally used and a large gripping surface or tab to allow ease of location in a purse and better grip.

The standard door height for mounting a latch at 40 inches from the floor is permissible if a lever handle is used. This would allow the wheelchair user to pull

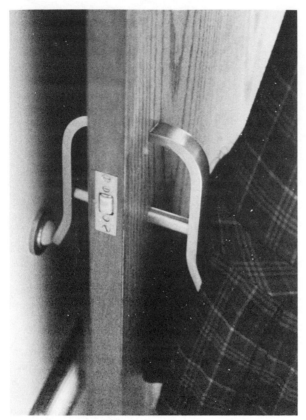

FIGURE 75
Inappropriate door handle. This fixed vertical handle is heavy, cold, and potentially dangerous. It will not give way when accidentally contacted by the torso or the head (as in the case of outward opening doors, which swing into the path of oncoming wheelchair users). (Photo: John Kelsey and Robert Steinbugler.)

downward on the handle and open the latch quite easily. Knobs with spherical or modified spherical gripping surfaces should be mounted at a lower height of 36 inches to allow the wheelchair user to exert force on the handle. This grip, as mentioned earlier, is not as desirable as the lever-type mechanism, but is more readily found in the marketplace.

The area around the latch and lock should be clear-ly marked off by a bright color or material contrasting to the door surface for ease of location.

FIXED AMBULATORY AIDS, HANDRAILS, AND SUPPORTS

Handrails in the corridor have been mentioned earlier. However, specifics regarding cross section and other specifications were not treated, nor was material given about the location of handrails in stairwells or on the steps in outside areas.

The grip portion of the handrail should have a cross section about 2¾ inches in diameter. In addition, a panel should project at the base of the graspable section with a cross section of 1 inch or more and have a rectilinear configuration. The depth of the panel should be 6 to 8 inches (Figure 32).

If a combination rail is used, there should be a 2 inch or more projection of the lower graspable section and the same projection for a panel. With a double rail for both ambulatory and wheelchair users, there would be no necessity for a panel on the upper rail.

The panel's function would be to prevent carts and other movable devices (including wheelchairs) from scrubbing the wall. The upper handrail should be mounted at 32 inches from the floor to the upper edge of the rail. A lower rail, if used, should be mounted at 26 inches for the same dimension.

There has been very effective use of lighting behind hand rails. This indirect lighting system is helpful in setting off the handrail and flooding the wall with light (photo) (see Figure 27).

Frequently, the handrail in a stairwell is not as carefully selected as the handrails in the hallway. Once again, the same cross section should be employed at the same height from the tread. Exterior grab rails, supports, and handrails must meet one additional design criterion that indoor versions do not: they must be impervious to weather conditions of varying temperatures and moisture. It is very tempting to use metal rails on the exterior of a building because of their resistance to climatic conditions. However, the feel and general esthetics in tactile quality of metal handrails leave a great deal to be desired. Metal handrails are also slippery when wet and electrically con-

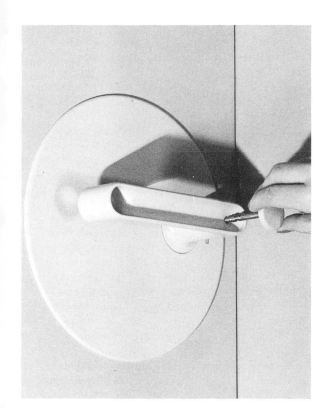

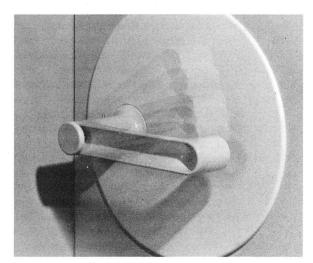

FIGURE 76

Lever–latch door handle for the manipulatively handicapped. Timothy Fauber and Paul Haninger developed the door-actuating mechanism shown here, which will give way under the force of an elbow, the torso or a severely impaired arm or hand because of the lever action. The extended handle provides ready purchase, unlike conventional cylindrical doorknobs. (Photo: Courtesy of ARMCO Steel Corporation.)

ductive. Metal handrails should be coated with either a plastic or vinyl coating.

SAFETY DEVICES AND FIRE DOORS

This subject area is one that is highly specified by codes and regulations. The devices employed, smoke detectors, sprinkler systems, alarm systems, and barriers, are subjected to frequent periodic inspection and requests for upgrading. There is constant reevaluation of safety devices in many states in nursing homes, and discussion of what systems are the best or what potential systems for the future might be like is outside the framework of this text. However, one device should be discussed because of its interference and impact, literally, upon the safety of the patient–resident.

The magnetically controlled fire door is hazardous to the safety of ambulatory and nonambulatory patient–residents. The doors close too fast. Anyone passing through the doorway or close enough for contact would be severely injured trying to get past the doors. It is difficult to specify for a complex electromechanical device of this kind, but there should be a mechanism provided that would make the door either remain open or open automatically when anyone was in its path. When passage of the person was completed, the door would then proceed to close again automatically.

One other aspect of emergency devices is their

general esthetics and visibility. Although they must be in plain view of anyone wishing to trigger off an alarm, nothing suggests institutional quality more than the safety devices currently used in nursing homes. There is a need for further consideration of the esthetics of safety devices, including the mechanical appendages such as alarm boxes, sprinklers, and other devices.

WALL FINISHES AND SURFACES

The walls in corridors take a great deal of abuse because of the traffic and variety of mobile devices used in these spaces. The wall surfaces in individual patient rooms take less abuse, but must function as display areas, therefore absorbing different kinds of abuse.

Corridor walls need much more intensive investigation in terms of use and abuse, and appropriate materials and surface treatments. Probably the least appropriate materials combination in corridors is the standard construction of drywall on wood stud framing. Regardless of whether or not this materials combination is painted or papered, the basic resilience of the drywall is too low and the material too permeable to allow for adequate preventive maintenance.

Brick, concrete block, and tile all have greater abilities to resist abuse, but they must be used judiciously because of safety and esthetic considerations. *No surface should be used which is so abrasive that it will cut, bruise, abrade, or otherwise injure patient–residents who are being pushed in wheelchairs or geriatric wheelchairs.* Often, the hands of these patient–residents are wrapped over the outside of the ambulatory device handles and are exposed to injury. Even rough-textured paints used on drywall can be too abrasive for use in this context.

On the other hand, slick textures that do not permit "purchase" or grasp for a dry hand should not be used. The reflectivity of these surfaces must also be considered very carefully to avoid glare.

It would seem that there is a spectrum of available materials which could potentially be used in the high traffic areas of the nursing home. On the one hand, these materials could be extremely durable but injurious because of abrasive surfaces. On the other, too

slick a surface presents little friction to stop falls, through the ability to achieve purchase from an outstretched hand, and excessive glare potential. Yet, in the middle of this spectrum, there are materials and combinations of materials and equipment (handrails, kickplates) that could perform adequately—and more than adequately in high use areas.

It is possible to use fire-rated drywall, cover the surface with a sprayed on coating, and cover this monolithic surface with either fiber glass fabric coverings or impregnated cloth wall coverings that will provide reasonable resilience and cleanability. However, these material combinations must be protected at the appropriate heights from abrasion from wheelchair hubs and at corners from a variety of possible abuses. This can only be accomplished through the use of horizontal extended barriers and kickplates at the base of the wall. If carpeting is utilized in the corridors, it may be possible to extend the carpet material up the wall or the kickplate approximately 6 inches to provide a uniform transition from floor to wall and reduce the number of different maintenance operations to clean the space (Figure 32).

Obviously, where an existing building is being redecorated or refurbished, there are a limited number of alternatives for upgrading. However, in new construction, a wider variety of possibilities are presented that might have exciting potential for future use.

The airplane passenger is acquainted with the interesting interior treatments of commercial aircraft. Much of the technology used in this context has a degree of application to high-use institutional structures.

The plastics industry has the capability to mold panels in a tremendous variety of sizes. The smallest vacuum-molding operation usually has the capacity to mold panels in 100- by 100-inch sections, drawn to a depth of 18 inches. It is within the realm of present technology to mold wall panels in a variety of plastic compounds, which could have excellent resilience, cleanability, low reflectivity, and appropriate texture for grasp, as well as molded in place handrails, kickplates, and light fixture implacements. The initial cost for setup of the molds and prototype runs would certainly be offset in the long run by the excellent maintenance and durability properties of the materials as well as possible fire resistance and sound attenuation characteristics.

In terms of esthetics, the plastics industry has the capacity to produce materials with virtually an infinite variety of visual appearances. The look of an interior might undergo so subtle a change that there is no apparent change in visual appearance at all. However, with some appropriate research and development, a new esthetic could be found that might not only be appropriate for the institution but also for the materials and their configuration. The drawback to research and development of building components manufactured in plastics is, of course, the diminishing supply of petroleum derivatives, from which the greater majority of plastics are derived, and their lack of fire retardancy. However, many substitutes are currently being investigated by the industry as replacements for compounds that may be in shorter supply in the coming years. Institutional building products research should move ahead with development in this area of materials, manufacturing, and design.

Floor surfaces are of great concern to most administrators and personnel in nursing homes. The great debate over whether carpeting or inlaid tile is superior continues. Because of the significant glare reduction possible with carpeted hallways and the advantages of safety and esthetics, carpeting should be chosen over hard floor coverings wherever and whenever possible. There is some discussion, but no formal evidence collected, that carpeting in corridors prevents some injuries due to falls where tiles would not be so preventative. There is also discussion, but no formal evidence, that there is less incontinence in nursing homes with carpeted floors than in nursing homes with tile floors. This would bear out the hypothesis that much incontinence is really a form of protest against institutionalization rather than a wholly physiological disorder.

The most serious drawback to the use of carpeting in nursing homes is the unfortunate physical properties of most undermats or backing materials. The largest number give off noxious fumes when they burn, even at slow rates of burn. The user of carpeting is forced to consider jute backings for carpets in order to prevent this characteristic occurrence during fire. There is also a heavy smoke produced during fire that impedes vision and seriously inhibits breathing. Jute backings do not produce these characteristics during fire, but they are more moisture absorbent. Therefore, when incontinence does occur, the jute backing will absorb it, retain the odors, and also rot after prolonged exposure. Again, more research and development should be directed at producing a carpet backing material that will not have the objectionable characteristics displayed by presently available products. A product of this type would not only have potential for institutional structures but also would enhance residential fire safety as well.

MATERIALS FOR DECOR AND IDENTIFICATION

There are an infinite variety of materials available for use as decorative surfacing materials for walls. Use of specific materials depends largely on taste and appropriateness within specific spaces. However, further consideration should be given to those materials which may be used to identify specific places for many patient–residents, especially those with advanced failing sight or the completely blind. An important characteristic of the materials chosen for an area is its texture, especially to the touch. Texture must be evaluated from the standpoints of both the visual aspect and the sense of touch.

Environments generally are far too overladen with visual as well as tactile textures. This presents a confusion to the eye as well as to the touch. Floor coverings, draperies, wood grains on doors, wall coverings, and the materials found on furnishings all contribute to the visual and tactile sense of a space. If the textures are not carefully combined, just as there should be a careful combination of color schemes, the result can be confusion, even for the well younger person. More importantly, there must be consideration given to the identity of a space as demarcated by textures. A great share of the patient–residents in a nursing home must rely on what they touch to clarify where they are.

There could be variations on the surfaces of handrails or tactile cues on doorsills and other locations so that spaces and locations could be identified. Today, many college campuses employ braille maps located around the grounds to help the blind and partially sighted to identify their location and to find other locations. There are many elevators in existence with braille identification markings to permit the blind to use the controls.

How many wall-mounted control panels for call buttons, temperature controls, bed controls, light controls, and other devices are designed to permit identification by texture? There are a multitude of areas in the nursing home where texture coding could be applied.

Color coding and graphic displays are also an important tool in aiding identification of location and space. However, color coding must be rated behind texture coding in terms of potential effectiveness for the identification of location and space. Colors can be perceived incorrectly or not seen as colors at all depending on a number of variable factors. The wide variety of perceptual difficulties of the aging eye account for some of the difficulty, but also the varying conditions of ambient and controlled artificial light will produce conditions under which colors effectively change from time to time.

To maximize effectiveness, color coding should be bold and striking, almost to excess. The wider the stripe or block of color the better for the most part. Written materials or signs should be bold, contrasting, and direct. White letters on black surfaces generally read better than the reverse, even for the normal eye. Pastalan's work at University of Michigan seems to bear this out for the aging eye as well (personal communication, 1975). Blue and green color combinations should be avoided because of their imperceptibility of difference to the aging eye. Color schemes in general should be conceived in the warm color range, and analogous schemes are preferable.

A redundancy of visual and tactile signals should be designed into a space so that there is a way of allowing spatial identification regardless of the sensory deprivation any one given patient-resident suffers. Where the handrail wavers or changes in surface treatment, there should also be a striking color design or readable sign in bold letters to help designate a space. It is not inconceivable that sound and smell stimuli

could be implanted at various locations to be a location descriptive device along with texture and color coding.

Visual and tactile identification schemes are not self-explanatory, however. A common mistake made when such systems are used is to believe that the patient-residents and others using the facility will recognize the cues and understand them as if they had intrinsic readability in relationship to the entire network of signals throughout the building. The staff must spend time with new patient-residents, orientating them to the building, access areas, and the coding system. This will ensure the workability of the system to the highest degree possible, and it will encourage the new patient-resident to take an interest in the building and in things other than his or her own problems.

WINDOW AND GLAZED SURFACES

Three aspects concerning windows installed in nursing homes are important factors to consider: (1) window placement, (2) window surface treatments, and (3) insulative qualities.

In the greatest majority of nursing homes, the window wall is directly opposite the entry area. Thus, patient-residents make a very abrupt transition from a low lighted condition in the corridor to an intensely lit condition inside the private room space.

With the physiological impairments in mind that afflict the sight of the greatest share of the patient-residents, identification of people in the space, seeing objects which may be directly in front of the person entering, and addressing other visual information is made extremely difficult in daylight conditions when there is no attempt to subdue the light in the space.

Window placement should be carefully considered in relation to the phenomena previously mentioned. It might be possible to locate the window on the exterior wall in such a way that penetration of the space by a patient-resident does not result in direct exposure to an intense glare situation. Another possibility is to locate the door and/or enclose the entry in such a way that there is more of a gradual transition into the space in terms of exposure to light. This type of design would allow for the slower adaptation time inherent in the aging eye. A combination of these two concepts of design could mean that the person penetrating the space would be facing diagonally into a given room, facing away from the light.

The treatment of a window surface, including both tinting or coloring the glass area and baffling the light through the use of screens, shields, blinds, and other devices, is very important in the determination of the quantity and quality of light inside the nursing home. Outside of the location of the building on a site in orientation to the sun, the treatment given to the glazed surfaces is of first importance in light control.

Generally speaking, reduction in the amount of glare produced by light in a space means reduction in the quantity of light available for seeing. However, natural lighting is far in excess of the quantity of light necessary for sight. In other words, all windows should be fitted with some means of reducing light quantities. Draperies are an obvious answer, but they are not always totally effective. Fully closed, the drapery screens off all visible activity in the external world. Vertical blinds mounted to the outside of a building structure as part of the architectural feature of the exterior can reduce light penetrating from one direction and still permit viewing of activity in another direction. Other devices exist as possibilities for both internal and external treatment of this kind. An important consideration is whether or not the control of the device employed can be provided to the patient–residents who use the space. Obviously, in a private room, a patient–resident should have control over the lighting as well as other aspects of the environment. In public space, another set of considerations may take precedence. The nature of activities going on, the number of people using the space, and the location of activities are a few of the considerations that dictate supervised control over lighting in public spaces.

Tinted glazing is available in a wide variety of types. One recent arrival in use in commercial architecture is copper-coated glass, which has high insulative characteristics as well as the quality of reducing light quantities. Amber glazing and smoked tinted glass have been available for many years. These two products lend a very definite cast or hue to the internal natural lighting of a building.

There are treatments available for glasses that cannot be produced commercially for glazing. Phototropic glass is a particular product that, through grinding, will become darker when the light striking the glass increases. Polarized glass will also reduce glare. However, both products would be extremely expensive to use in commercial glazing.

SOUND-ATTENUATING DEVICES

One predominant problem in a nursing home is the amount of background noise found throughout any given facility. The reverse can also be the case, so little sound, such a hushed quiet, that the building is more like a tomb than a place for living. In the first instance, careful consideration must be given to the dampening of sound in some locations; in the latter, serious questions should be raised about the institutional atmosphere of the place plus the use of drugs. Too much sound is an easier problem to handle than too little sound.

The designer and administrator should be careful not to screen out helpful sounds. Noises emanating from an activity room, lounge, or dining room serve as locators of the space, just as signs and coding devices locate spaces. However, once inside public spaces, the background noise can be excessive. For the aging, there is difficulty in discriminating conversation from the general "white" noise heard throughout a space. While the entrance way might funnel noise into the corridor so that the space can be located, the interior surround should be quieted through acoustical treatments and sound-attenuating devices.

Generally speaking, treating a space for acoustical control means considering the construction materials used in the building process in terms of their acoustical properties. Building engineers generally have competence in this domain, and should be able to advise the builder or developer of the facility as to the treatment of a space with specific construction materials.

Sound-attenuating devices are those implements

used after construction to dampen sound in a space. This might include carpeting, fabric, or woven type wall hangings, fibrous panels hung from the ceiling, and even mechanical devices that are available to counter background noise.

One typical problem found in the public spaces in the nursing home is the cathedral ceiling, which reflects sound. Even moderately noisy spaces of this type can be bothersome to the aging patient–resident who has hearing difficulties, because conversations from other locations in the space may seem to be emanating from his or her companions, and there is a struggle to understand and respond.

One of the easiest methods of moderating the sound in a space of this type is to hang banners, fabric hangings, and acoustical panels at the arch of the ceiling. This will cut the amount of sound re-flected to some degree. The walls may also be treated so that they too will dampen the sound otherwise being reflected around the room.

The secondary treatment of wall and ceiling areas with various devices has a twofold benefit. First, the intent is to dampen sound, and this can be accomplished with appropriate selections of materials. The second benefit is of equal importance; spaces will be enriched with color, texture, and other visual stimuli, which will add greatly to the richness of a space.

REFERENCE

ARMCO Steel Corporation. Designing to Accommodate the Handicapped. ARMCO Steel Student Design Program, Middletown, Ohio, 1974.

RECOMMENDATIONS FOR UTENSILS, DINNERWARE, TOOLS, PACKAGING, AND CONSUMER PRODUCTS

The common ground for recommendations in this area of design is that each group of specific items requires particular dexterities of hand–eye coordination when in use. Also, in addition to the combined effect of visual and manipulative dexterities, the singular aspects of being seen and graspability should also be considered. The aging patient–resident sitting in a dining room with a meal to be eaten, must see the meal, the vessels and containers of that meal, and the implements to be used. The various items must be grasped and held firmly to be used. Finally, the distances and positions must be perceived correctly to be moved the appropriate way or used correctly to obtain desired results–eye–hand coordination. All these functional considerations are involved in the proper design and selection of table settings, consumer products, and packaging.

One way of referring to this area of specification for nursing homes is attention to detail. These small things can often be very disconcerting and the very elements that frustrate and depress the patient–resident about his or her infirmities. Often, embarrassment results in a turning away from the offerings and activities of the facility, and there is an unfortunate alienation.

To some degree, and sometimes to a great degree, all people at some time are handicapped. Either through disabling sickness or injury, normal pregnancy, or just physiological and/or psychological happenstance, every person experiences less than optimum possible performance. While this may be true for the majority, the majority also believes that they will regain optimum performance. The momentary incapacitation is tolerable because recovery is in sight. For many of the aging, this is not the case. The important concept about their condition is that they must retain the least incapacitation for as long as possible.

Therefore, the small products that surround patient–residents in nursing homes are either subtle prosthetic devices meant to defer further disability, or they are less than subtle reminders of failing health.

Since the mealtime activity is so very important in numerous ways, unfortunate choices of table settings will have a very pronounced effect on the perception of self in the nursing home setting.

Dinnerware should be chosen that will contrast with the background tablecloths or table surfaces. All too often the choice is a white on white combination that is very difficult to see, especially at the noontime meal in high natural lighting. Plates and other crockery should either be in the warm or earth-tone color range or have a distinct pattern. The edge of the plate should be bordered so that the periphery can be seen easily. The top surface of the dinnerware should be lifted from the surface of the table so that there is an offset, permitting a shadow to form at the base from any source of lighting. Another important feature not easily found among the standard offerings in dinnerware is an upturn on the edge of the plates permitting the diner to force food onto forks and spoons by moving it against the edge. Plate collars can be purchased. However, these devices have the look of specialized equipment and are clumsy.

Glassware should not be completely clear. Smoked or colored glass should be used; again, there should be a ring around the top so that the edge can be easily seen and located.

Television sets, radios, clasps on pocket books, and the like, all require fairly high levels of ability to perceive the necessary control, manipulative procedure, and operation. Generally, the larger the surface area of the control, the easier it will be to manipulate. Unfortunately, many electronics companies in recent years have tended to reduce the size of controls instead of enlarging them.

One very useful development is the use of sliding controls on stereo equipment in particular. Although there is still no effort to enlarge the surface of the control for adequate grasp, the movement and positioning of the control are very easy to manage and to understand. This contrasts with dial-type controls, which are difficult to read prior to operation and then difficult to understand in terms of correct direction for manipulation.

Two important directions in manufacturing have yet to be explored by either designers of products and architectural hardware or producers of goods: (1) the design and fabrication of adequate specialized equipment and products for nursing home and other health related facility settings, and (2) the design and fabrication of products and equipment suitable for the handicapped population as well as the well.

Since this culture is surrounded with electronic gear and this way of things seems not to be diminishing,

more thought must be given to the production of this equipment with more suitable controlling elements for a wider range of the population. This development would actually be in the best interests of the manufacturing community. As population trends change the proportion of elderly to younger people, there is evident need to create products more in line with the human factors commensurate with aging (Figures 74 and 77).

The shape of salt and pepper shakers, creamers, and other items found on the typical dinner table should be graspable, identifiable, and interpretable (which end pours?). Obviously, condiments are not going to be placed on the table in the greatest percentage of nursing homes. However, in facilities related to nursing homes these specifications are important.

There are no good flatware settings for the elderly patient-resident of nursing homes. Knives, forks, and spoons are basically designed from the standpoint of esthetics with the basic functions very traditionally applied. To be sure, this is a most difficult design problem. A very detailed study of the manipulative difficulties of the institutionalized population should be undertaken to generate good flatware, as well as other products that depend on manual dexterity, grasp, and control. Again, specialized flatware is often clumsy and a distortion of the standard variety of utensils. Confronted with special tools, the aging patient-resident is confronted with a loss of control.

Those who choose these accoutrements of the physical environment have a greater problem than there would seem to be at first glance. Choosing those things that look nice is not necessarily the best approach. However, confronted with even the minimal information presented here the task multiplies in difficulty.

Products and packaging present the same kinds of problems to the administrator and staff, and also to the patient-resident, as dinnerware settings and flatware. The most important human factor is the ability to perceive and manipulate an infinite variety of small items.

While designing and manufacturing of products and equipment should be sympathetic with the real needs of the population as a whole, there remains the problem of selection for those who must purchase equip-

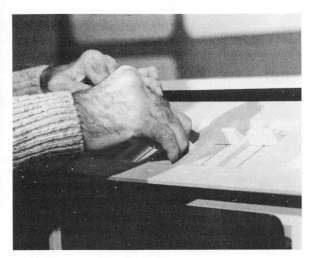

FIGURE 77
Arthritic moving specially designed television controls. (Photo: Courtesy of ARMCO Steel Corporation.)

ment for the nursing home on a *continual* basis. By the time the building has been completed and the interior has been finished, the services of the designers usually have been long since terminated. After the first five-year operating period, replacement becomes the most important continuing "design" function. This is a design function because every choice made will in some way affect the overall environment, its use, and the general esthetic quality.

There are two important design phases in nursing home facility programming: (1) the building phase, and (2) the replacement and refurbishing phase. The programming aspects of these two phases will be discussed in the final chapter, but there are some extremely important decisions about design that merit discussion at this point. First, the designers of the building should be retained through the construction phase and the equipment-selection phase. Designers have reference materials at their disposal that administrators and staff people do not have, and it is important to minimize the mistakes that can be made through a poor initial selection process. An experienced architect in the building of nursing homes will know which kinds of equip-

ment have worked in the past, and this is valuable knowledge to have.

With regard to the replacement process, it may be unnecessary to retain a designer every time a new television set is purchased, but it is possible to set up a program of replacement with a qualified interior designer or industrial designer. Most qualified architects can recommend other designers who would be able to help in this selection process. Another possibility is that where a facility is large enough, with a great replacement problem on a continuing basis, a designer should be retained as a staff member to help in the selection of equipment and products. In a very short period of time, this person will acquire a personal working knowledge of the facility, its staff, and its patient–residents. This feeling for the environment could be valuable in the long run. It could be the responsibility of this designer to make certain that any selection is in keeping with the overall objectives of care and rehabilitation of the facility as a whole.

At first, this idea seems extravagant. However, there is no question that a tremendous variety of poor choices of equipment have cost hundreds of thousands of dollars after buildings have been completed. Administrators and developers should remember that only about 3 percent of the cost of a facility is in the initial construction phase. The remainder will be spent on staffing, programs, and refurbishing. The cost of one additional staff member could be worth thousands in savings over the program life of the building.

Another facet of this person's responsibility would be to coordinate with the patient–residents so that their input can contribute to the design process. The ultimate users of all the products and equipment should share in the responsibility on a continuing basis as well.

PACKAGING

One of the most serious problems in nursing homes is accessibility to containers and packaging. For the more independent elderly, drug containers present accessibility problems, especially since the advent of child-protective devices a few years ago. Once again, the specific problems of manipulation of these types of containers should be studied, and specific proposals for special designs for the aging population should be rendered (Steinbugler et al., 1971).

Labeling is also a great problem. Many elderly adults have several medications in their possession at the same time, and because the package labels are so similar, there can be confusion. The industry should establish a common system of labeling drugs for easy identification and legibility.

While the nursing home patient–resident is usually not in possession of drugs which he or she takes at individual discretion, these populations are confronted with a wide variety of gift packaging, food packaging, and other containers that require high degrees of dexterity and perceptual skill. Virtually no packaging commonly available has graphics designed to be read or perceived and understood by anyone other than the most able. In many cases, packaging is very esthetically sophisticated in order to capture a highly developed and sensitive respondent. In general, this nation has so much tradition and experience with advertising that it has become highly attuned to this avenue of communication. As a result, the message projected by a package or by the items themselves is less important than the means by which it is communicated. This is art without reason; a triumph of design esthetics over human comprehension.

In this area of design and its impact upon the special groups of consumers, there will be little progress until a massive change in attitudes is developed. Manufacturers, advertising people, distributors, and others involved in the total network of product creation and packaging must become aware of the shortcomings of the system they have created.

For those who buy and choose, there can only be frustration over the lack of appropriate designs. However, experiences can be shared; and if responsible people exchange information about good design and where it might be found, change can occur.

Establishing a program of packaging and containerization surveillance would be helpful in nursing homes and other health-related facilities for the elderly. Criteria should be established by the staff, which would include specifications on labeling of all packages that enter, ease of opening, and extraction of contents. Developing a system of labels including large print and color coding for a given facility would be helpful for the staff and the patient–residents. Providing information to families and to other visitors about packaging and labeling would also be helpful.

REFERENCE

Steinbugler, R., K. Brandhorst, E. Stott, M. Barton, S. Marko, and B. Wegener. "Project: Design Containers Suitable for Holding Medicines and Other Dangerous Substances Found in the Household, and Make the Containers Childproof." *Human Ecology Forum*, 1, no. 1 (1971).

PART **V**

CONCLUSION

PROPOSAL
FOR RESEARCH
AND DEVELOPMENT

A decade ago, the automobile companies in this country utilized an interesting device to acquaint the public with new developments in design and research. They used vehicles of the "future" to project advances in the state of the art of automotive design. In actuality, these vehicles were far from futuristic; they were conglomerations of a variety of engineering advances and package changes, which were very much a feasible set of alternatives to be implemented on production vehicles. However, by introducing these changes to the public in one package, they became more acceptable when they appeared on the production vehicles a short time later.

Similarly, much that is known about the design of institutional settings for the elderly cannot surface in "production" facilities. As has been shown in this text, there are technologies, psychological and sociological concepts, design ideas for products and equipment, and other exploratory changes that might be experimented with and demonstrated in an appropriate "experimental" facility. In this way, new ideas would gain exposure when and if they proved feasible, and the obviously feasible ideas would have quick demonstrated worthiness for immediate application.

A proposal was submitted recently by a leading architect to an international panel of research-orientated professionals along the lines of the experimental facility described. While the proposal submitted was extremely ambitious, the seeds of research and development were clearly embodied in that proposal. If the concept were to be developed to its fullest extent, attention would need to be given to every facet of the programming of the most sophisticated nursing home facility. The physical environment would be only the formal manifestation of the overall scheme of care. The trend toward geriatric centers has a great deal of viability because no elderly person regardless of infirmity or level of incapacity can be excluded. This concept also allows for progressive rehabilitation or possible deterioration, both of which are possible among this population.

Perhaps the most important decision at the onset would be *to plan and design from the inside out*. This means that focusing on the person—the patient-resident in his or her own world in his or her own space—is where the project must begin.

Another important aspect of the planning to be dealt with at the beginning stages of the project would be the inclusion of community programs for those who reside in the facility as well as elderly who would be brought into the facility, attracted by the variety of things to do and people to meet and share with. How much attachment to the community with regard to what levels of physical capability is an unanswered question and worthy of exploration. It has tremendous ramifications for the entire rehabilitation and socialization program.

With respect to the physical design of the physical plant, there are numerous possibilities that should be explored. After all the social and medical planning has taken place, there are experiments with building development that could be exciting in terms of potential for other projects. The escalating costs of construction necessitate exploration of the concept of industrialized building in the institutional field. It has been shown in other fields, hotel–motel construction and to some degree public housing, that agglomerating the total dwelling unit requirement and relating this need to industrialized construction can save money through mass buying of materials and equipment. A stock unit that has been proved through trial and experimentation would be usable in other projects as well. It is also possible that, through the development of an experimental project, the costs of setting up a special plant for industrializing the construction of institutional structures could be amortized and other buildings established at further cost reductions (Carreiro and Mensch, 1971).

The usual fear of architects and other designers is that repetition of units will result in a sameness and duplication of initial mistakes. However, it has been shown that industrialization ensures as much if not more variety as do traditional building methods. In fact, there is very little variety among the architecture of modern large-population nursing homes. With the exception of external facades, the internal arrangement is usually dictated by the economy of minimizing extraneous space to ensure maximized room exposure to outer window walls. It is a wonder that after millions of double-loaded corridor arrangements duplicated over the past 20 years there is any need to talk of the necessity for architectural variety.

Variety, to be achieved, must come through a conscious effort to ensure that the physiological and psychological needs of the patient–residents are met rather than through any dependence upon design creativity. This traditional approach has consistently failed in the past, and mistakes are constantly duplicated because of an insistence that there is an inalienable right maintained by the designer to explore his own mind, find his own way, and originate an idea. This process has lead inexorably to rediscovery of the wheel almost every time.

There is so much room for improvement, through a conscientious effort to improve the lot of those who must remain in the nursing home, that to impose personal conceptions about design is an affrontery to the population who must live with the designer's mistakes.

If architecture as a profession must come to grips with different ways from the traditional to design effective buildings for the aging, the other design professions and manufacturers of institutional equipment and furnishings must do it for the first time. There are practically no good pieces of institutional furnishing on the market today, designed with the patient–resident's needs as a criteria base. Geriatric chairs are designed to accommodate the staff who need to restrain someone. The comfort of the chair is secondary. Fixed seating, as has been discussed, is primarily designed with incontinence as a dominant criterion.

The input of manufacturers to an extended project of this kind would be beneficial to the elderly as well as to the manufacturers. There is a need to know whether or not ideas about extended seating prove out. This experimentation would be better conducted in a controlled environment than on a hit or miss basis through market research or buyer responses in the marketplace. Prototypes of all kinds could be developed, which then could be examined thoroughly over a long period of time, modified and improved if need be, and finally marketed if they show decided improvement.

It is hard to conceive of flaws in an experimental facility of this kind. With regard to proving out design concepts, many product and equipment designs have been around for 20 or more years and will continue to be marketed because there is presently no research and development to improve designs. Reliance on evolution in the application of new technology and ideas generated in other countries has been the major mechanism through which change has occurred. This is not a sufficient basis to create change in products as rapidly as change should occur for the populations in various settings who are older now and are growing older in increasing numbers. The design and construction of an experimental facility should accelerate the process of change.

Clearly, there are significant issues to be dealt with concerning the use of human subjects in such an undertaking, especially those people who may not be able to understand the nature of their involvement. Very careful consideration would have to be given to the control of the setting and the free will of the participants.

Conversely there has been tremendous experimentation with elderly subjects for many years—and much of the experimentation has been of a far more questionable nature than the more unobtrusive involvement with changes in the physical setting: the use of LSD on terminal patients, Skinnerian motivational and behavioral modification experiments, the early stages of reality therapy, and the like. Therefore, while the use of human subjects would be an issue, along with other important issues, there is evidence that the cooperation of professionals in the broad field of gerontology can be found and many elderly would be willing to participate.

The most serious question of all is whether financial support for such an undertaking is available. Clearly, no governmental source has a specific mandate in the area of research and development outside of the Defense Department. The research currently being financed by the federal government is not orientated in the direction of creating physical hardware. Changing the priorities of these agencies would prove frustrating and counterproductive to other important research and demonstration that is of benefit to the elderly.

Probably the most productive avenue is to agglomerate a consortia of industrial, management, consultative, and building enterprises to cooperate by giving technical, material, financial, and administrative assistance in the development of one project or a combination of research and development projects. While the information would be made public, there would be a decided advantage in lead time for an industrial manufacturing cooperator who participated from the very beginning of the project. By pulling together a large number of cooperators, the cost to any one of the participants would be small for the gain in having participated. In fact, by building a broad base of support for the project, no one concern could dominate, while everyone could potentially gain.

To effect the proper control of such an undertaking, there would need to be involvement of perhaps one or more of the universities where gerontology is a major concern. While the location of the project need not necessarily be in the proximity of an educational institution, there should be access to the facility by academic personnel who wish to be involved in such a project. The specific arrangements for such accessibility would need further clarification, just as would the specific roles of contributors. However, there is an obvious need for a consortia of the academic and research interests with business and market interests in such a project.

To mount such an effort, a six-phase program would seem to be in order:

1. Identification of the interested parties for cooperation in a research and development effort.
2. Formulation of a proposal for specific research and development assignments to be carried out by various cooperators.
3. Gathering of support from both contributors to the proposal and others who may wish only peripheral or outside involvement.
4. Realization of research and development goals on the part of contributors, coordinated through one central administrative source, and then the synthesis of various developments at one or more sites.
5. Evaluation and monitoring of the facility(s) by research control groups and experimentation with a variety of social and educational programs in conjunction with medical and rehabilitation programs on a longitudinal basis.
6. Systematic reporting of results, publication of advances, and distribution of information over time on the progress of the project.

This project would be, like so many other proposals, an ambitious undertaking. However, in this country there is no other means by which design development can take place, except through minimal efforts within industry.

There is no question that, if such an undertaking could be mounted at all, the time involved for even partial results would be measured in years. Perhaps five years would be necessary in order to reach a point where developments stemming from technological and other forms of research could be combined in one or more pieces of architecture on any given site. Five more years might pass before the results of evaluation can be shown. However, while the project is in progress, a tremendous amount would be learned that could be applied directly to production projects—even without evaluation. The process itself would be fruitful because new experiences and associations would be happening on a continual basis.

An obvious alternative to this approach is piecemeal research and development on a scattered basis whereby individual projects are supported without combination in one or more controlled settings. While this alternative is less productive, it would advance the state of the art of design for the elderly, but with a tremendous increase in time. The question central to this issue is whether or not the time is not now critical to begin solving important design problems?

REFERENCE

Carreiro, Joseph, and Steven Mensch. *Building Blocks: Design Potentials and Constraints.* Ithaca, N.Y.: Center for Urban Development Research, Cornell University, 1971.

EPILOGUE:
COMMENTS FROM
A DESIGN ADVOCATE

The reader of this text should be aware that the content is the product of a thinking process which is strongly biased toward design. There is an inclination on the part of designers to assume that design, especially the design of physical objects and physical environments, is a path to the improvement of man's lot. To be sure, there is much about the whole system of health care, and in particular the nursing home concept, that is wrong for man and antithetical to rehabilitation after illness regardless of design.

Many argue that the management of nursing homes is not what it should be or that a health care system which, by and large, is profit motivated can never be truly humanistic. Many argue that the aging are really socially deprived over and above everything else, and so improvement of the social context of the environment for the aging is paramount. Still others insist that a good dose of money liberally administered directly to the aging population would do the trick.

There is merit in all these directions, but just as many counterarguments that impede any one concept about health care from coming to the fore— excepting the present situation. Indeed, the profit– nonprofit argument rages, and the nonprofit sector

seems to be gaining strength, even statistically in numbers of beds provided across the nation.

In lieu of the arguments and counterarguments about the most effective way to deliver health care, it seems important to state several significant points that have a relationship to the concept of building and designing nursing homes:

1. The United States needs a well-balanced approach to caring for its older citizens with an emphasis on maintaining independence of living, choice of environment, and choice of social surroundings.
2. There should be far more experimentation with programs that stress maintenance of life in the home and less reliance on institutional settings as a be-all and end-all.
3. Nursing homes are meant to support the needs of the chronically ill aged who need 24-hour surveillance and rehabilitation to the highest possible level of health and independence.
4. Multitype, multiphased health care programs stressing maintenance of the elderly in the community will not hurt the nursing home concept. With an expanding older population, the need

for upgrading the current nursing home stock, and improvements in health care financial support mechanisms, there will actually be an overload on the current bed supply. No informed planners, government officials, designers, or nursing home administrators actually believe that the nursing home is endangered by alternatives to nursing home care.

5. Older people should not be forced to live any-where—especially in nursing homes. As stated, the open nursing home has as many ways of getting out as it has for getting in. There should be an emphasis on rehabilitation to leave rather than on rehabilitation to maintain.

6. Design of environments, any environments for any population, is not seen as a panacea for all the problems related to the general social, psycholog-ical, and physiological aspects of environment. However, where an environment can be designed to be supportive rather than unsupportive of its population, there should be every effort to design environments with support as a premise.

7. The intensive medical atmosphere of nursing homes has not been effective as a means to rehabilitation of chronically ill aged population. It would seem that rehabilitation to levels of self-maintenance should be the goal in spite of the problems this en-tails. Where possible, elderly people who need as-sistance beyond the nursing home should be raised to this level of independence, discharged, and then monitored and assisted within the community structure. A more intensive social and stimulating environment is seen as a means to making the transition between acute care and the home.

8. Many older people will live out their life in the nursing home. In some nursing homes, the major-ity of the patients will die there. However, as this text has emphasized, this phase of living—not dying—is developmental in nature, and every living person in the nursing home needs to strive for as much living as is possible.

Many of the arguments that send out word-missiles use the same vocabulary in their warheads in spite of the fact that the arguments are opposing. "Quality care" is one such warhead, but the definition of this little word combination means so many different things to different people that it is hard to tell who is talking about what. There are obvious inferences about quality care in this text. However, to a physi-cian, quality care means the delivery of the highest level of medical assistance that is possible within given circumstances. This text is no argument against that idea. Rather it is an attempt to ask the question: is the delivery of quality medical care always synon-ymous with providing lots of nurses, drugs, medical equipment, and periodic inspections by health of-ficials? The answer must be no, because that is the situation presently and it is not working totally ef-fectively. Another way of stating the problem is that there is no way to legislate effective care of people. Attitudes toward care and attitudes about people must be supportive to begin with.

In this respect, there is much about the design process and the culmination of that process which addresses this point. Architects know that a building can be designed in two ways: one way is to let codes predominate and to do nothing more than satisfy the regulations and those officials who administer them; the second way is to constantly strive to formulate concepts that are oriented to the popula-tion served by the building first, and then address codes after the concept has been formed. When this motivation enters the design process, there can be an assurance that "quality" is uppermost in the minds of the design team. Also, as has been stated through-out this text, the physical environmental complex is the most controllable component of the entire environmental complex surrounding everyone. Better training programs can and should be developed for staff personnel, their administrators should be up-graded, and means should be found to reinforce the social framework involving the elderly. However, the changes from these important facets of care will be long in coming and in many ways difficult to per-ceive. The physical environment is a visible piece of evidence of changing attitudes and the concerns of all who serve within them.

It should also be noted here that the author does not subscribe to the often heard cliché that nursing homes are representative of our failure to deal effec-tively with the medical, psychological, and social problems of our country; in other words, if all else fails—put them in a nursing home. While the specialized chronic care health facility is inappropriate for many of the elderly who may be in them now, there will always be a need for the nursing home, regardless of how they are designated and no matter what jargon or argot is manufactured to disguise them.

From another standpoint, however, the general thrust of design for as long as it has been practiced in conjunction with technology has been to segment specific populations for which products have been designed. The elderly have been excluded from this process. Thus, special efforts are necessary to create designs in housing and special products to fill the gap. This is perhaps the greatest failing of the technological–manufacturing sector of this society. What is particularly ironic is that the marketability of attuning the productive capacities of modern industry to the needs of the elderly has been proved to be extremely sound economically and potentially lucrative. Yet the whole focus of American consumer product producers has been myopically directed away from the elderly. It has been shown statistically in almost every category of business market research that now and in the future the buying power and the area of greatest need rests with the older people of the United States.

Designers and industrialists alike must address themselves to a wider spread of needs. Products designed in this country must be directed at a market made up of adults from the years of 17 to 80, rather than to one solely under 25 or only half the total range. Those who do direct attention in this way can be assured of growth; those who do not will surely experience decline.

Here, again, design of the physical environment and the artifacts which are part of that environment make up an important part of the quality of life. An "inclusive" philosophy about design would help the elderly remain within their own environments, living independently longer than the current "exclusionary" philosophy.

A pressing issue with regard to effective design of environments for the elderly, and any other age group for that matter, is the need for *more* use of design expertise in the first place. As previously stated, at crucial points in the design process, designers are often not employed or utilized. Architects are often used to generate the plans of a facility, but not given the chance to consult on the detailing phase of interior architecture or the furnishing selections. Industrial designers, a group acquainted with human engineering principles to as great a degree as any design specialists, are currently "underemployed" in the design of furnishings, equipment, tools, and other products selected for nursing home environments. In a manner of speaking, the trouble with the design of most environments is that they are totally *undesigned* in the first place.

There never will be pat answers to design problems. Surely, efficiency and economics may dictate that certain specific answers to problems will repeat and be duplicated. However, there can be no design cookbook. Design by its very nature defies formulas. Thus, the administrator or staff member who selects furnishings or sets the specification for the interiors of buildings is not in a position to know how to "relate" various elements, even when the elements are the very best selections.

Another possibility to be investigated is that of retaining designers either on the staff of a nursing home facility or as consultants over the life span of the building or at critical phases in redesign and refurbishing. There is the evident possibility that design expertise on board on a continuous basis could be a tremendous cost saving to facility managers owing to the knowledge of products and furnishings the designer possesses.

This book is an attempt to show how many possibilities exist for change and the utilization of design expertise. It is important to state that leaving out the use of design expertise at critical periods of change, as well as in new construction, is a great mistake (Koncelik, 1973).

It seems that change is so possible and the effort to produce change so near as to be almost painfully close. Everyone who touches the environment for the elderly has a design input to make of a kind. The designer has that special input of integration of physical elements which cannot be excluded. It has been said by Dr. Philip Land, the designer–inventor of the marvelous Polaroid Land cameras, that if a problem can be stated clearly, it can be solved. In terms of the nearness of the solution of design problems related to nursing homes, perhaps this book has been successful in a partial way in providing the necessary articulation about these special environments so that better design can evolve. Finally coming to grips with the problem of design for the aging means, in the long run, solving everyone's problems. Too many have waited too long.

REFERENCE

Koncelik, Joseph A. "Site Planning, Structural Design, Interior Design and Furnishings; Part II." In *Non-Profit Homes for the Aging: Planning, Development and Programming*. Los Angeles, Calif.: University of Southern California, 1973.

(Photo: David O. Watkins.)

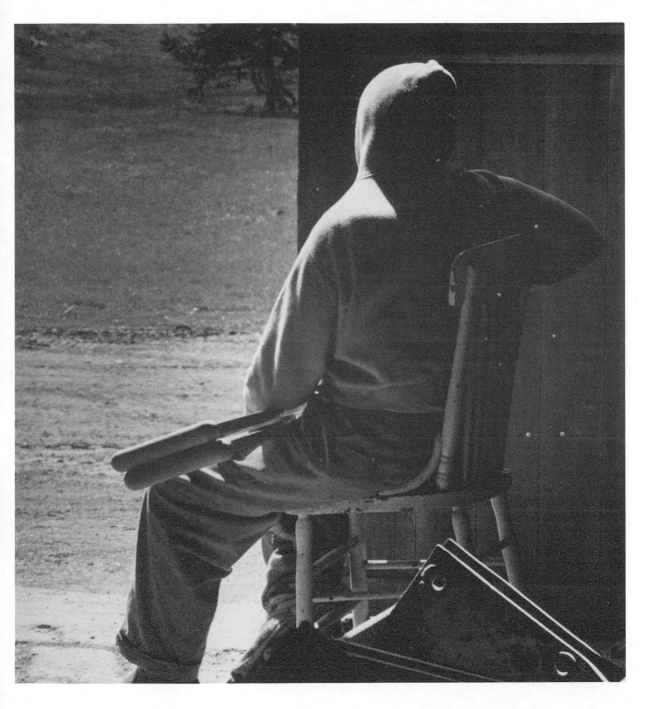

INDEX